Tendons - Trauma, Inflammation, Degeneration, and Treatment

Edited by Nahum Rosenberg

Published in London, United Kingdom

Tendons - Trauma, Inflammation, Degeneration, and Treatment
http://dx.doi.org/10.5772/intechopen.104180
Edited by Nahum Rosenberg

Contributors
Bruno Silvestrini, Mauro Silvestrini, Shen Liu, Rui Zhang, Yanhao Li, Rong Bao, Qinglin Kang, John Christian Parsaoran Butarbutar, Nahum Rosenberg

First published in London, United Kingdom, 2023 by IntechOpen
IntechOpen is the global imprint of INTECHOPEN LIMITED, registered in England and Wales, registration number: 11086078, 5 Princes Gate Court, London, SW7 2QJ, United Kingdom

British Library Cataloguing-in-Publication Data
A catalogue record for this book is available from the British Library

Additional hard and PDF copies can be obtained from orders@intechopen.com

Tendons - Trauma, Inflammation, Degeneration, and Treatment
Edited by Nahum Rosenberg
p. cm.
Print ISBN 978-1-83768-185-3
Online ISBN 978-1-83768-186-0
eBook (PDF) ISBN 978-1-83768-187-7

Meet the editor

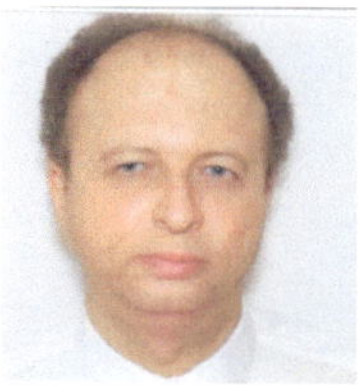

Nahum Rosenberg, MD, Ph.D., MOrthop, MBA, FRCS, is an orthopedic consultant surgeon with more than 30 years of experience. He graduated with an MD from the Faculty of Medicine, Technion Israel Institute of Technology (Technion-IIT) in 1990. He obtained a Ph.D. from the University of Portsmouth, UK. He completed his residency in orthopedic surgery at Rambam Medical Center, Israel, in 1997. Dr. Rosenberg has devoted a great deal of time to basic research, which helped him earn a MOrthop (Distinct) degree from Tel Aviv University, Israel, in 1996. Between 1998 and 1999, he was appointed as a Nuffield Fellow in orthopedic surgery at Oxford University, UK. He was also a clinical fellow at Mercy Private Hospital, in Australia. In 2002, he was hired by the University of Nottingham, UK, as a clinical fellow in orthopedic surgery (upper limb surgery). In 2018, he completed an MBA in Biomedicine at the College of Management Academic Studies, in Israel. Dr. Rosenberg has worked as a senior orthopedic surgeon at the Rambam Health Care Campus since 2003. In 2007, he was appointed assistant clinical professor in the Faculty of Medicine, Technion-IIT. Dr. Rosenberg actively participates on the editorial boards of ten journals on orthopedic surgery. He served on the International Society of Arthroscopy, Knee Surgery, and Orthopedic Sports Medicine's (ISAKOS) Shoulder Committee. He has 80 peer-reviewed scientific articles, 5 books, and 150 presentations at international scientific meetings to his credit.

Contents

Preface

Tendons are the biological and mechanical interface between muscles and bones. Their physiological role is to transfer the force of the muscle contraction to joint movements. As such, tendons have semi-elastic properties due to their connective tissue content and therefore are prone to inflammatory, degenerative, and structural failure that can cause disabling effects, primarily pain, and impaired joint function.

Tendon-related disabilities (tendinopathies) can significantly impact a person's daily functions. Tendinopathies can result from various causes, such as acute injury, systemic disease, or overuse. The following are the most prevalent causes of disabling pathology related to tendons:

- Tendinitis: This is an inflammation of the tendon, usually caused by overuse and repetitive strain or systemic inflammatory disease. The most common anatomic sites prone to tendinitis are the shoulder, elbow, wrist, knee, and ankle. The clinical manifestations of tendinitis involve pain, swelling, and limited mobility.

- Tendinosis: This is a chronic degeneration of the tendon that occurs following microtrauma. It can also be caused by aging or other medical conditions. Tendinosis can cause pain and weakness in the affected areas.

- Tear or separation: This can be caused by a sudden injury or by overuse. Tendon rupture can result in severe pain, swelling, and loss of function in the affected limb.

- Tenosynovitis: This is inflammation of the synovial membrane surrounding the tendon. Tenosynovitis can result in pain, swelling, and limited mobility. It is most prevalent in the hand and wrist.

This book highlights recent advances in the current understanding of the mechanical and inflammatory structural pathologies involving the tendons. It also discusses the biochemical characteristics and mechanics of tendons and examines traumatic and degenerative causes (e.g., acute tears and microtrauma) of impairment. Furthermore, it presents pharmacological approaches for inflammatory conditions involving tendons.

Nahum Rosenberg
Specialists Center,
National Insurance Institute,
Haifa, Israel

Section 1

Introduction

Chapter 1

Introductory Chapter: Tendons – Trauma, Inflammation, Degeneration, and Treatment

Nahum Rosenberg

1. Introduction

> *"When a joint becomes painful, swollen, and inflamed, it is impossible not to consider the ligaments and tendons, as they are the immediate cause of these symptoms."*
> *Citation attributed to Hippocrates.*

Tendons are specialized connective tissues essential for transferring forces from muscle contraction to the bones, enabling joint movement and mobility. Due to the semi-stiff nature of the tendons, forces may be effectively transferred from the muscle to the bone. Tendons' mechanical strength makes it possible to withstand mechanical forces.

The collagen fibers within the tendon have a very well-organized structure, which accounts for their strength. On the other hand, tendons display some viscoelastic activity that is dependent on the rate and length of loading. This characteristic enables tendons to adjust over time to variations in mechanical loading. As a result, tendons resist structural failure even under repeated strain. Its resistance to fatigue results from the tendon cells' capacity to repair and remodel the tendon according to its stress–strain characteristics, expressed by the stress–strain curve (**Figure 1**) [1, 2]. This curve determines the tendon's stiffness and toughness and present the maximum force the tendon can withstand before failing. A tendon's structural and mechanical characteristics may alter over time due to degeneration or damage, according to changes in the stress–strain curve.

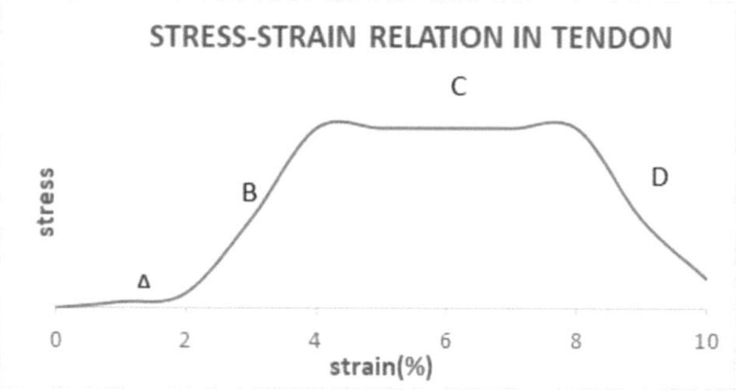

Figure 1.
The stress–strain curve of a tendon – A simplified schematic representation.

These biomechanical features are made possible by the peculiar structure of tendons. A sheath of connective tissue (such as the endotenon) surrounds the collagen fiber bundles that make up tendons at the microscopic level, where they are arranged into fascicles. The endotenon has a vascular and nerve supply that allows the tendon to receive nutrients and react to external stimuli.

The basic structural element of tendons is collagen fibers (the primary type is type I collagen). The parallel bundles they form give the tendon its strength and stiffness. Moreover, tendons include elastin fibers that provide some semi-flexibility and allow them to stretch slightly in response to stress (toe region on the stress–strain curve). Tenocytes, which are fibroblasts in the tendon tissue, is crucial to preserving the tendon's form and functionality. The collagen and elastic fibers of the tendon are produced and maintained by these cells. In addition, tenocytes can adapt the tendon to changes prompted by the stresses of a contracting muscle because of their mechanosensing characteristics.

A. Toe region – the tendon can withstand stress of low magnitude with minimal strain (up to ~2%). This region is due to the straightening and reorientation of the crimped collagen fibers within the tendon. B: Linear region – elastic deformation (a strain of ~2–4%) when the tendon returns to its original shape once the stress is removed. This region is due to the stretching of the collagen fibers within the tendon. C: Microscopic failure region- the tendon beyond the plastic deformation (a strain of ~4–8%) and incapable of returning to its original shape once the stress is removed. This region is due to the rupture of the collagen fibers within the tendon. D: Total structural rupture of the tendon (a strain above ~8%).

The distinctive structure of tendons is created by type I collagen, which makes long, thin fibers grouped in parallel bundles. Other forms of collagen, such as type III collagen, are also in minor quantities in the tendon tissue. The tendon's structure and function are supported by type III collagen, which is present in lesser levels and is less rigid than type I collagen.

As a result, the tendon is made up of fascicles that are packed with multiple parallel collagen fibers. A matrix of proteoglycans and glycosaminoglycans holds these fibers together while also acting as a shock absorber and lubricant thanks to the presence of synovia-like material. Collagen molecules repeating units are arranged staggered to form the collagen fibers. The tensile strength of the tendon is provided by this arrangement [3, 4].

The myotendinous junction is created at the tendon-muscle interface, where the collagen fibers of the tendon are continuous with the muscle fibers.

The fibrocartilaginous enthesis is created at the tendon–bone junction, where the collagen fibers of the bone and the tendon are continuous. The enthesis is a unique area with numerous discrete zones with various compositions and architecture. A highly organized structure called the fibrocartilaginous enthesis enables effective force transmission from the tendon to the bone. The multiple zones of the enthesis are designed to withstand the various mechanical stresses at the interface, such as compressive forces in the highly mineralized fibrocartilage zone and tensile forces in the tendon zone due to the well-aligned collagen fibers.

Tendon collagen content varies according to environmental and endogenous factors, such as age, systemic conditions, and specific anatomical location.

Thus tendon is a complex structure dependent on material and biochemical factors; therefore, it might be susceptible to mechanical failure, acute or degenerative, and pathological inflammatory conditions of connective tissue disorders. This makes the tendon a source of numerous disabling conditions expressed by pain and movement disorders [5].

This book addresses and discusses several unique and clinically important tendons-related issues. This text should be an important information source for clinicians treating musculoskeletal pathology.

Author details

Nahum Rosenberg
Specialists Center, National Insurance Institute, Haifa, Israel

*Address all correspondence to: nahumrosenebrg@hotmail.com

References

[1] Robi K, Jakob N, Matevz K, Matjaz V. Chapter 2. The physiology of sports injuries and repair processes. In: Hamlin M, Draper N, Kathiravel Y, editors. Current Issues in Sports and Exercise Medicine. London, UK: Intech Open; 2013. pp. 43-86. DOI: 10.5772/54234

[2] Maganaris CN, Chatzistergos P, Reeves ND, Narici MV. Sec. Exercise Physiology. Frontiers in Physiology. 28 Feb 2017;**8**:1-11. DOI: 10.3389/fphys.2017.00091

[3] Thorpe CT, Screen HRC. Tendon structure and composition. In: Ackermann P, Hart D, editors. Metabolic Influences on Risk for Tendon Disorders. Advances in Experimental Medicine and Biology. Vol. 920. Cham: Springer; 2016. DOI: 10.1007/978-3-319-33943-6_1

[4] Kannus P. Structure of the tendon connective tissue. Scandinavian Journal of Medicine & Science in Sports. 2000;**10**(6):312-320. DOI: 10.1034/j.1600-0838.2000.010006312.x

[5] Zabrzyński J, Łapaj Ł, Paczesny Ł, Zabrzyńska A, Grzanka D. Tendon - function-related structure, simple healing process and mysterious ageing. Folia Morphologica. 2018;**77**(3):416-427. DOI: 10.5603/FM.a2018.0006. Epub 2018 Jan 18

Section 2

Mechanical Aspects

Chapter 2

Tendon Injury Following Strenuous Activity: (Acute, Repetitive, and Chronic)

Nahum Rosenberg

Abstract

Tendon biomechanics are governed by tendon structure. The collagen fibers' "uncrimping effect," which transforms their mutually nonparallel orientation to parallel in response to external force, underlies the range of tendon elasticity. The Golgi tendon organs control tendon proprioception. The mechanosensing proprioception may help to some extent protect the mechanical integrity of the tendon; in degenerative tendons, it could be expressed by pain. The tendon's intrinsic structure may fail when the acute, chronic, or recurrent external load exceeds the tendon's structural and mechanical resistance. The most significant factor leading to tendon rupture is excessive load, either acute or repetitive. When aging or a chronic illness is present, the magnitude of the excessive load is reduced.

Keywords: tendon, stress, strain, golgi tendon organs, proprioception

1. Introduction

Regular exercise is necessary to keep our body parts healthy, and tendons are no exception. Tendinopathy involves damage and inflammation of certain tendons due to chronic overuse or acute injury.

Tendons' structure defines tendon biomechanics. When the environmental and mechanical loads exceed the maximal strain resistance of the tendon, it will structurally fail, and an eventual rupture of the tendon will occur. For this purpose, the damaging mechanical strain may be due to a high acute extensive load or lower repetitive loads that build up the critical extensive stress on the tendon. These two patterns distinguish between acute tendon structural failure and structural failure due to overuse loads, that is, acute tendon rupture vs. rupture following microtrauma to the tendon.

2. Pathophysiology

The tendon elasticity range is based on the "uncrimping effect" of the collagen fibers that change their mutual nonparallel orientation to parallel following external

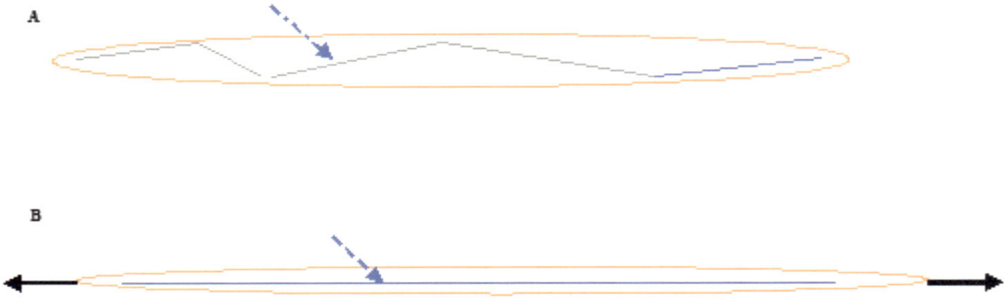

Figure 1.
A simplistic representation of the "uncrimping effect" in the tendon. A: Relaxed tendon with the nonparallel orientation of the collagen fibrils (dashed arrow). B: Stretched tendon by external loads (solid arrows). The collagen fibrils in a parallel orientation allow the elastic tendon elongation.

load (**Figure 1**) [1]. Beyond the elasticity range, with rising stress on the tendon, the integrity of the tendon is based on its collagen fiber content. In contrast, the latter integrity depends on its biochemical characteristics, which depend on age and/or systemic diseases. Therefore, the tendon tangent modulus, which represents the non-elastic range of stress effect on the tendon, depends on age and a specific biochemical environment following systemic illness [2].

The more prevalent systemic conditions that predispose to tendon degeneration are connective tissue diseases (Rheumatoid arthritis, Systemic Lupus Erythematosus, etc.), Sarcoidosis, inherited diseases involving damaged collagen metabolism (Ehlers–Danlos syndrome, Marfan syndrome, and homocystinuria), and more [3].

Still, mechanical excessive load, either acute or repetitive, is the most important cause of tendon rupture. Naturally, the magnitude of the excessive load is lower when exists the factor of age or systemic illness.

The main protective mechanism from the excessive load damaging effect is the proprioception of load buildup on the tendon and pain.

The Golgi tendon organs govern the tendon proprioception. These are mechanosensing structures encapsulating afferent axons in the tendon–muscle interface, therefore interconnecting between force-generating muscle and neural protective feedback [3]. The Golgi tendon organs are thought to interrelate with muscle spindles in governing muscle-generated force, while limb kinesthesia determines the safe extent of limb movement.

3. Clinical manifestations

Therefore, the physiological limb movement is governed by the feedback of mechanosensors in muscle-tendon "force generators." This type of biofeedback of movement causes, for example, the "paradox effect" of higher mean angular acceleration in the abduction of a nondominant arm during intentional limb rise (**Figure 2**) [4], although the force generation potential of the dominant arm is higher (**Figure 3**) [5].

A more exact physiologic requirement can explain this phenomenon when the dominant limb sacrifices the force demand in favor of precision, and this is orchestrated by the proprioceptive feedback from mechanosensors in tendons and muscles.

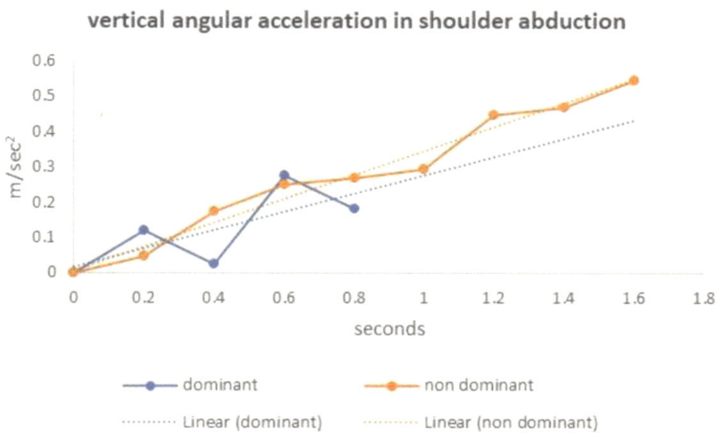

Figure 2.
Example of vertical acceleration during abduction in an adult individual without known shoulder pathology. The linear trendline of movement of the nondominant arm has a higher rate of force buildup in comparison to a dominant limb (linear slope of 0.34 vs. 0.26).

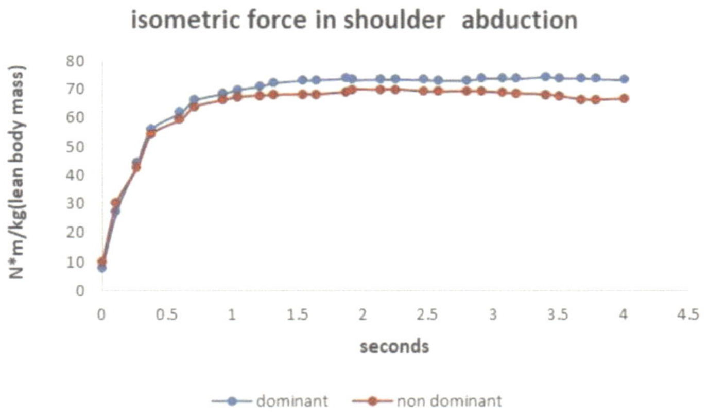

Figure 3.
Example of a force moment buildup during shoulder abduction in an adult individual without known shoulder pathology. The maximal moment in the dominant arm is higher than in a nondominant limb.

Therefore, the tendon's mechanical integrity, determined by its intrinsic properties, may be protected to some extent by the mechanosensing proprioception and might fail when the external load, acute or chronic repetitive, exceeds the latter properties of the tendon.

The pain from the structurally degenerated tendon might have a protective role in further tendon damage, even by lower loads, but this assumption should be further clarified.

Therefore the maximal isometric moment around the joint is significantly diminished, mostly due to pain, when intrinsic tendon damage exists, even without a complete tendon tear (**Figure 4**) [6].

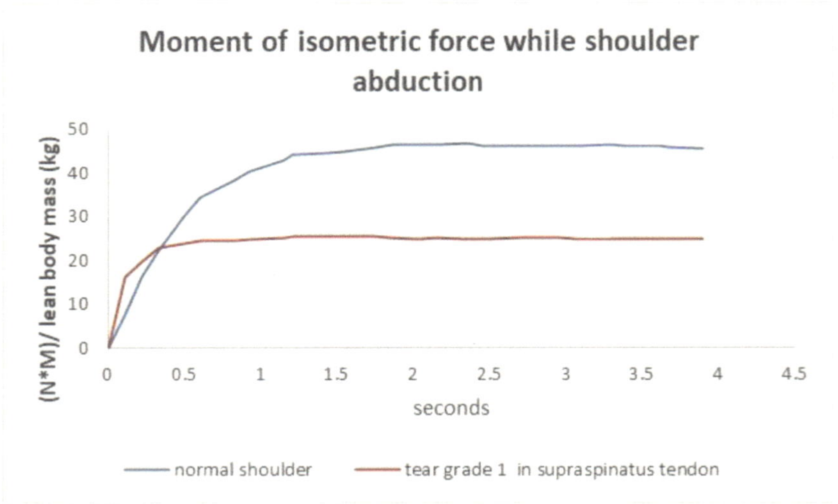

Figure 4.
Example of a force moment buildup during shoulder abduction in adult individuals with and without intrinsic tendon damage. The maximal moment in the normal arm is twice higher than in the case of the rotator cuff with a small degenerative tear.

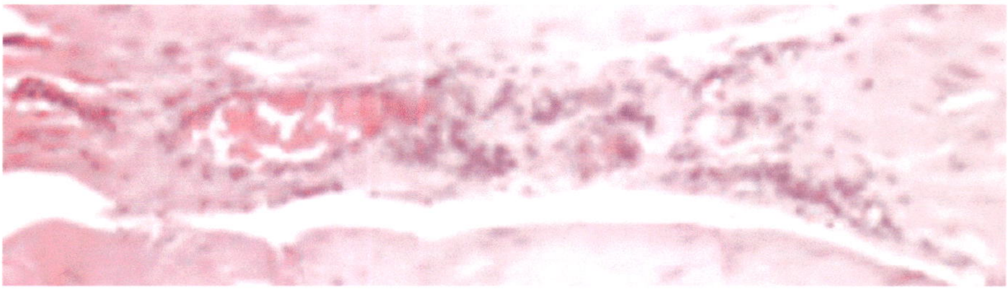

Figure 5.
Degenerative fibrotic tissue in the common extensor origin characteristic of lateral epicondylitis in the elbow. Myxomatous expansion is seen around blood vessels.

A good example of this phenomenon of significant functional impairment is a painful elbow and arm due to lateral epicondylitis, although, In this situation, pain is generated by a relatively small area of tendon degeneration in the common extensor origin at the lateral epicondyle of the distal humerus (**Figure 5**) [7].

Furthermore, the kinematics of the joint, while physiological movement, when a painful tendon is involved, appears to be mechanically inferior to the normal joint, even when the continuity of the degenerative tendon is preserved (**Figure 6**).

Therefore, pain from the shoulder tendinopathy following an acute not physiological load or due to repetitive load, with subsequential microtrauma to the tendon, might be etiologically considered as a protective mechanism from further tendon damage because the pain intensity does not always relate to the extension of the structural impairment in the tendon. Moreover, it is apparent that usually, although the structural damage in the degenerative tendon does not justify mechanical interference with the transfer of force from the contracting muscle to joint movement, still the force generated during joint movement is reduced, and the only causative reason to this impairment is pain originating from the degenerative tendon.

DOI: http://dx.doi.org/10.5772/intechopen.110550

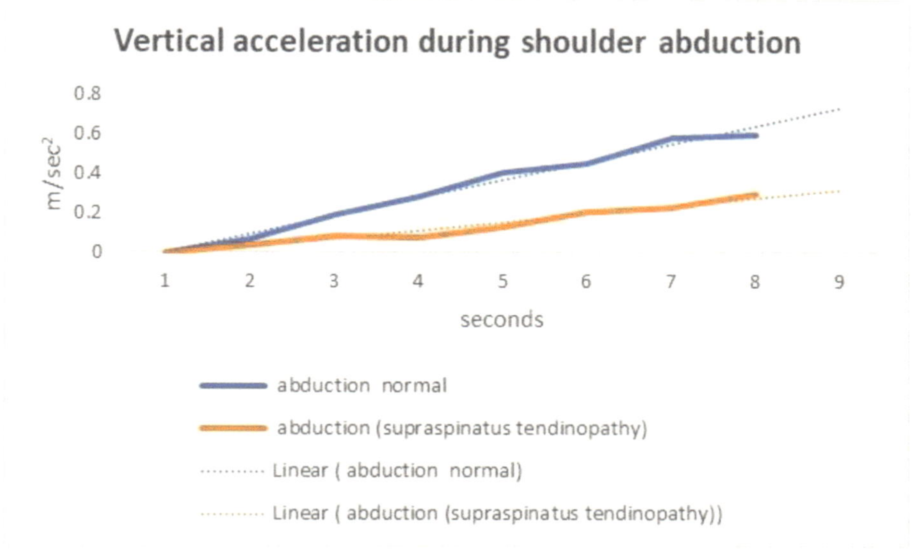

Figure 6.
Example of a vertical force buildup (expressed by acceleration) during shoulder abduction during an unresisted intentional shoulder movement in adult individuals with and without intrinsic tendon damage. The maximal moment in the normal arm is twice higher than in the case of the rotator cuff with a small degenerative tear. The linear trendline of movement in the individual without rotator cuff tendon pathology has a twice higher rate of force buildup compared to the individual with supraspinatus tendinopathy (linear slope of 0.09 vs. 0.04).

This observation should be taken into consideration in the clinical setup when the patients' complaints of pain generated by the tendinopathy are seldom related to the extent of the intrinsic damage of the involved tendon.

4. Prospective

Pain is a subjective complaint, and its quantification is usually obtained by functional self-assessment scores and related to the visual analog scale (VAS). Currently, there is no widespread agreement on the correlation between pain severity and joint impairment due to tendinopathy. Such clinical correlation is imperative for the rational decisions of treatment and the grading of the disability. The main obstacle is the decision on the clinical program related to subjective complaints versus objectively relatively non-extensive tissue damage. Meaning that the standardization of patient disability evaluation in the context of tendinopathy is currently insufficient.

For this type of clinical standardization, the ability to quantify the subjective level of pain is of basic importance [8]. Unfortunately, such an objective method of pain quantization does not exist in clinical use.

Aiming to overcome the difficulty of getting objective measurements of the subjective pain sensation, there is an ongoing research attempt to quantify the pain intensity by the composite algorithms of objective data processing [9]. For this purpose, the main clinical data readily available in the everyday clinical setup may include electrophysiologic and mechanical measurements.

There is experimental evidence that processing such multimodal signals, that is, pulse rate, blood pressure, electroencephalogram, and recording eye movement and facial expression, might provide a basis for a reliable grading of pain level [10].

Thus if the combined data processing methods of pain quantization are available for clinical use in the physician's office setup, it will be possible to evaluate the morbidity caused by tendinopathy, not only on its structural extent but on a more reliable basis of the level of joint impairment due to pain. This study can give an efficient tool and guide for the decision- making, medical and surgical treatment, and disability evaluation related to tendon injury or tendinopathy.

Author details

Nahum Rosenberg
Specialists Center, National Insurance Institute, Haifa, Israel

*Address all correspondence to: nahumrosenebrg@hotmail.com

References

[1] Franchi M, Fini M, Quaranta M, et al. Crimp morphology in relaxed and stretched rat Achilles tendon. Journal of Anatomy. 2007;**210**:1-7

[2] Zuskov A, Freedman BR, Gordon JA, Sarver JJ, Buckley MR, Soslowsky LJ. Tendon biomechanics and crimp properties following fatigue loading are influenced by tendon type and age in mice. Journal of Orthopedic Research. 2020;**38**(1):36-42. DOI: 10.1002/jor.24407

[3] Järvinen M, Józsa L, Kannus P, Järvinen TL, Kvist M, Leadbetter W. Histopathological findings in chronic tendon disorders. Scandinavian Journal of Medicine & Science in Sports. 1997;**7**(2):86-95. DOI: 10.1111/j.1600-0838.1997.tb00124.x

[4] Jee H, Park J. Comparative analyses of the dominant and non-dominant upper limbs during the abduction and adduction motions. Iranian Journal of Public Health. 2019;**48**(10):1768-1776

[5] Chezar A, Berkovitch Y, Haddad M, Keren Y, Soudry M, Rosenberg N. Normal isometric strength of rotatorcuff muscles in adults. Bone Joint Research. 2013;**2**(10):214-219. DOI: 10.1302/2046-3758.210.2000202. PMID: 24100165; PMCID: PMC3792443

[6] Rosenberg N. Rotator cuff isometric strength across the life span in a normal population and in patients with rotator cuff pathology. Chapter 2. In: Imhoff A, Savoie F, editors. Rotator Cuff across the Life Span. Berlin: Springer Nature; 2019. pp. 11-17

[7] Rosenberg N, Henderson I. Surgical treatment of resistant lateral epicondylitis. Follow-up study of 19 patients after excision, release and repair of proximal common extensor tendon origin. Archives of Orthopaedic and Trauma Surgery. 2002;**122**:514-517

[8] Titan A, Andarawis-Puri N. Tendinopathy: Investigating the intersection of clinical and animal research to identify progress and hurdles in the field. JBJS Review. 2016;**4**(10):01874474. DOI: 10.2106/JBJS.RVW.15.00088

[9] Cowen R, Stasiowska MK, Laycock H, Bantel C. Assessing pain objectively: The use of physiological markers. Anaesthesia. 2015;**70**(7):828-847. DOI: 10.1111/anae.13018

[10] Lin Y, Xiao Y, Wang L, Guo Y, Zhu W, Dalip B, et al. Experimental exploration of objective human pain assessment using multimodal sensing signals. Frontiers in Neuroscience. 2022;**16**:831627. DOI: 10.3389/fnins.2022.831627

Section 3

Biochemical Aspects

Chapter 3

Tendon Adhesion and Novel Solutions

Shen Liu, Qinglin Kang, Rui Zhang, Yanhao Li and Rong Bao

Abstract

Tendon adhesion refers to the development of fibrotic tissue accumulation between injured tendon and the surrounding tissue, which usually happens as complications after surgical intervention for tendinopathies or traumatic rupture of tendon, resulting in undesired outcomes in the aspects of mechanical properties and functionality. Researches and understanding of tendon adhesion indicate that the process is related to the dominance of extrinsic tendon healing, with important factors such as inflammatory response, cell transference, certain growth factors, mistakenly stimulated signaling pathways and infection, and overdriving tendon remodeling. Taken the advantage of advanced material science and biochemistry, novel biomimetic materials have gradually emerged and been revealed to obtain satisfying antiadhesion capabilities. Taken the advantage of advanced material science and biochemistry, novel strategies, including hydrogels, nanoparticles, nanofibrous membranes, and substitutions for tendon and peritendinous apparatus, have gradually emerged and been revealed to obtain satisfying anti-adhesion capability solely or as drug delivery platforms. Although most of these results are currently limited *in vitro* or in animal models, future modification of these biosynthetic materials will help gain better mechanical properties and biocompatibility for clinical application. The establishment of next-generation delivery platforms against tendon adhesion requires the crosstalk among multiple fields.

Keywords: tendon adhesion, mechanism, countermeasure, advanced material, drug delivery system, future direction

1. Introduction

Tendons are dense connective tissue extending from muscles, which travel across joints to transmit force and produce motion. Although tendons possess remarkable tensile strength that can tolerate large force generated from muscle contraction, they are susceptible to damages caused by chronic overuse tendinopathies and traumatic rupture [1, 2]. It is noted that lacerated tendons cannot undergo spontaneous healing and surgical procedures are often required [3–5]. Conventional reconstruction techniques, including suturing, grafting, and synthetic prothesis replacement, however, are unfortunately associated with postoperative adhesion formation between surrounding tissue and the injured site, which results in undesired outcomes in the aspects of mechanical properties and range of motions.

With a better understanding of peritendinous adhesion, it is widely accepted that the process is related to the dominance of extrinsic tendon healing. To illustrate, the early inflammatory response and external fibroblast invasion are mainly responsible for the promoted tendon adhesion [6–9]. Intrinsic factors of tendons, including low cellularity and metabolic activity, along with limited blood supply, also lead to a slow rate of tendon healing and remodeling, which increases tendency of re-rupture and hampering outcomes [10, 11].

Diverse strategies have been applied to overcome this clinical challenge. When anti-inflammatory drugs, antiadhesion growth factors, and certain genes that inhibit peritendinous adhesion have shown satisfactory outcomes in experimental studies, solely using these degradable molecules still face many limitations including swift inactivity, uncontrolled release, and toxicity before clinical translation. Besides, although physical barriers such as silk, silica gel and gold foil promote tendon gliding when wrapping around the injured site, with little biodegradability, these materials may inhibit intrinsic healing and cause body rejection, eventually leading to tendon necrosis and reoperation [12, 13]. Hence, current researchers have shifted their attention towards combinatory approaches, combatting tendon adhesion through loading different pharmaceutics and biologics into three-dimensional scaffolds, which were fabricated via various techniques including cryo-drying, solvent casting, gas foaming, braiding, and tissue engineering [14]. These scaffolds enable critical functions such as cell adhesion, proliferation, differentiation, and response to extracellular signals, while important issues still need to be discussed and improved. The scaffold should generally allow sufficient vascularization and interchange of nutrients and wastes, which is essential for tendon healing, while abnormal immune reactions should not be risen by the artificial scaffold [15, 16]. Additionally, adequate mechanical strength of the scaffold is also of vital importance to support tendon repair, mechanical load and gliding [17]. Besides, cargoes of the scaffolds should have promising effects on preventing peritendinous adhesion through alleviating inflammatory response, restricting unusual fibrogenesis, accelerating intrinsic healing, and promoting lubrication [18, 19]. In recent years, biosynthetic materials, including hydrogels, nanoparticles, nanofibrous membranes have gained wide attention for tendon adhesion prevention and have shown marvelous effects *ex* and *in vivo* [14, 20, 21]. At the same time, the advancement of biological materials and their derivations such as amnion, pericardium, and tendon sheath also shed light on strategies of tendon reconstruction and adhesion prevention [22–27]. However, low accessibility of the resources, low productivity of the advanced biochemical products, and unknown biocompatibility to human body curbed their application to clinical usage [14, 20].

This chapter provides a comprehensive discussion of the current understanding of the mechanisms through which tendon adhesion is supposed to form, and identifies the pearls and pitfalls of the advanced biomaterials in preventing tendon adhesion.

2. Tendon structure and mechanisms of peritendinous adhesion

2.1 Tendon structure and composition

Tendon is composed of water (55–70% of whole tendon) and collagen (60–85% of dry weight) [28]. Type I collagen is the primary collagen in tendon, which accounts for 90% and the rest are type III, V and XI [29, 30]. Tendon also contains glycoproteins, cells and so on [31, 32].

Tendon is arranged orderly in a hierarchical manner which includes six levels: collagen molecule, pentafibril, collagen fibril, collagen fiber, fascicle and whole tendon. The basic unit of tendon is collagen molecule, five of which are bound together to form pentafibrils (also called microfibrils). Pentafibrils pack together to form collagen fibrils [33, 34].

In tendon, collagen fibrils are the unit of collagen fibers that aggregate to form fascicle with diameters ranging from 50 to 300 μm. A connective tissue, interfascicular matrix (IFM), is bound around the fascicles which is also the elemental structure of tendon. Moreover, the tendon is covered by the epitenon which is connected with IFM.

2.2 Tendon regeneration and repair

Tendon healing is a long period including three phases: inflammatory (days 1 to 7), fibroblastic (days 3 to 14), and remodeling (beyond day 10). Once tendon is injured, both external and internal cells are recruited and proliferated surrounding the injury site such as macrophage outside and tenocytes inside. After 3 days, the collagen is deposited to form extracellular matrix at the injury site, especially collagen type III. Then collagen type III is turned to be type I during the remodeling phase to heal the wounded tendon. However, the biomechanical strength of the healed tendon cannot reach as good as the one of the uninjured (**Figure 1**) [12, 35].

2.3 Factors affecting tendon adhesion

2.3.1 Inflammation

An acute inflammatory response to tendon rupture site is initiated lasting for 3 to 7 days [7, 8, 36]. In the initiation stage after tendon injury, the gene expression of pro-inflammatory cytokines significantly ascends attributed to recruitment of neutrophils, macrophages, and monocytes [37–39]. The inflammatory storm response to defect site after tendon injury is extensively considered as contribution to tendon adhesion formation and confusing matrix degradation, both of which are attributed to substantial up-regulation of inflammatory factors simulated by activated fibroblasts and matrix degradation [40, 41]. Besides, inflammation-mediated increased exudation and aggravation of fibrin leakage also lead to promotion of tendon adhesion formation. Therefore, spatially and temporally further understanding and adjustment to inflammatory response to tendon adhesion during the whole process of tendon healing will be far more crucial in inhibition of tendon adhesion formation.

2.3.2 Cell transference

Tendon healing includes the effect of both internal and external cells [42]. During the phase of inflammation, external cells play an important role in the adult tendon [43]. Neutrophils are recruited into the injury site in the first 24 h. Few minutes later, monocytes and macrophages reach, and macrophages become the dominant cell population instead of neutrophils after 24 h. Macrophages can be categorized into two main types: classically activated (M1) or alternatively activated (M2). Generally, M1 refers to the function of proinflammation, while M2 is considered an element of

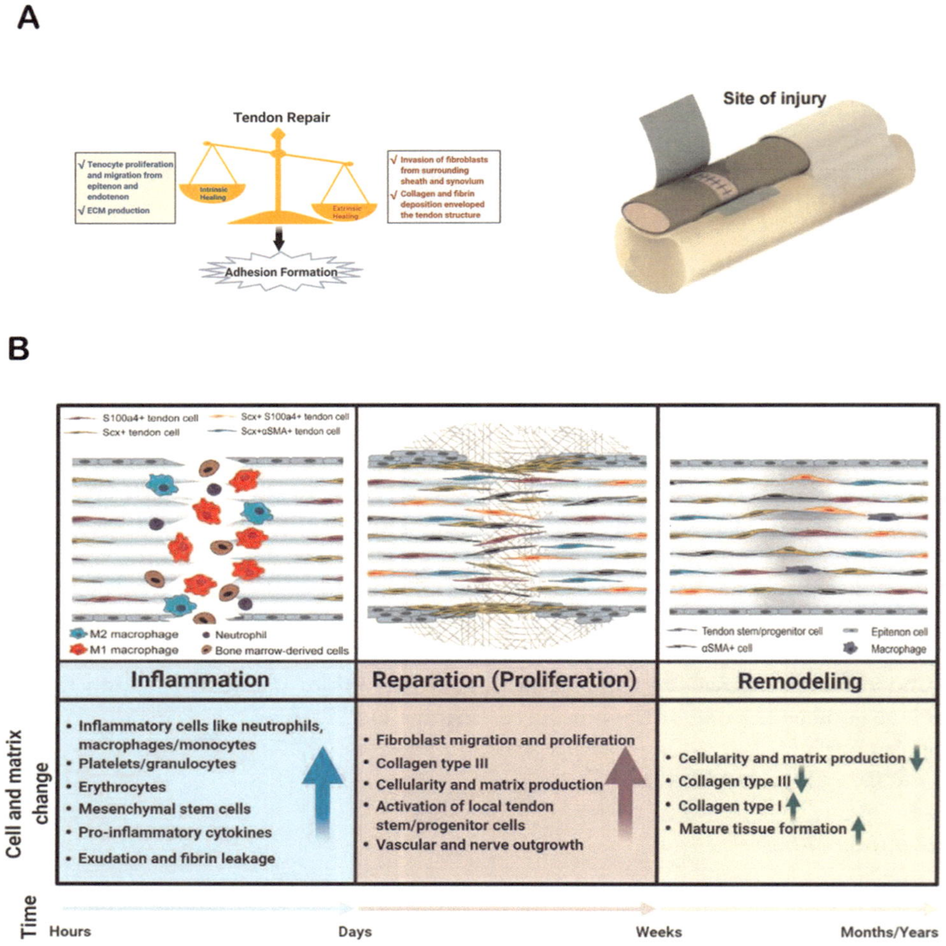

Figure 1.
(A) Peritendinous adhesion formation due to the unbalance between the intrinsic and extrinsic tendon healing, where antiadhesion materials are placed and function locally. (B) the key cellular and matrix changes and duration of three tendon injury repair phases (inflammation, reparation, and remodeling).

antiinflammatory response [44]. There are also other cell populations contacted with the phase of initial tendon injury such as T cells and mast cells [45, 46].

When it comes to the proliferative phase, the obvious character is the deposit of collagen type III in the injury site released by cells, especially fibroblasts. To begin with, it is the epitenon cells that proliferate. Both canine and murine models can be seen that the layer of epitenon become thicker in the early phase of proliferation [6, 47]. Epitenon cells can release more fibronectin than tendon itself, especially in the scar of injury site [9]. Nearly 2 days after injury, fibroblasts were recruited and proliferate rapidly, while the origin of fibroblasts remains unclear. Recently, researchers have identified a few different populations of resident tendon stem/progenitor cells involved in tendon healing, including cells from tendon fascicles, epitenon, and perivascular cells [48–53].

After 10 days, there are fewer cells in the scar which is called the remodeling phase. Generally, the scar is finally replaced by organ-specific cell populations such as bones. However, scar in the tendon is partly replaced. The decrease of scleraxis basic helix–loop–helix transcription factor positive tendon cells may attribute to this phenomenon [54]. Moreover, the external cells such as inflammatory cells and myofibroblasts also play an essential role, but the explicit mechanism remains to discover [55, 56].

2.3.3 Growth factors

Generally, it is considered that GFs mainly work on proliferation phase overlapping the inflammation phase [7]. GFs, including transforming growth factor-beta (TGF-β), vascular endothelial growth factor (VEGF), basic fibroblast growth factor (bFGF), platelet-derived growth factor (PDGF), bone morphogenetic proteins-12, -13, and -14 (BMPs) also known as growth and differentiation factors-5, -6, and -7 (GDFs) respectively and insulin-like growth factor-1 (IGF-1) has been extensively authenticated their existence during different phases of tendon healing and regeneration process, and their significant roles have been widely studied [21, 57–60]. TGF-β1 is an isoform of TGF-β with multifunction, which is widely demonstrated as main cytokine for tendon adhesion formation [61, 62]. VEGF, bFGF, and PDGF have been demonstrated to promote tendon healing by intensifying mesenchymal stem cells (MSCs) proliferation and differentiation to tenogenic lineages, increasing vascularization and ascending biomechanical strength after tendon regeneration [63–66]. BMPs have been shown great induction force to tenogenic differentiation of MSCs as well as necessity to the regeneration of tenocytes, especially BMP-14 has been utilized to initiate tenogenic lineage of adipose-derived stem cells (ASCs), and it is widely demonstrated its high efficiency of pro-differentiation when associated with ASCs [67–72]. However, BMP-14 has also been reported its an additional benefit of tendon adhesion resistance during tendon healing [58, 73]. Furthermore, whether the final production of BMPs activation is tenogenic or osteogenic lineage relies not only on the isoform of BMPs but also the type of biomechanical stimulation [74, 75]. IGF-1 has been proved to stimulate regeneration and tenogenic lineage differentiation of ASCs, however, the recent question regarding the practical usage of IGF-1 in tendon healing is whether IGF-1 acts independently or cooperates under the guideline of growth factors for single use of IGF-1 presented abominable outcomes in tendinopathic human patellar tendon [76–79]. Therefore, in-depth understanding of the multifarious roles of GFs not only by themselves but also in synergy with others will help us better understand tendon adhesion formation and anchor efficient therapeutic targets.

2.3.4 Signaling pathways

Inflammation, cell recruitment, and growth factors provide new insights of mechanism of tendon adhesion formation, and these factors may produce marked effects under the specific guidelines of signaling transduction process concatenating above three. After tendon injury, the tendon biomechanical changes including but not limited to loss of collagen fiber tension, primary cilium deformation and nuclear deformation initiate the pathology reaction by accumulation of specific molecular messengers such as ions or cytokines [80]. Inflammation is the primary pathology reaction raised up by a certain signaling pathway. The nuclear factor-kappa B (NF-κB) signaling pathway is involved at the initial stage of inflammation during the tendon healing. It is located in the cytoplasm and enters the nucleus after activation playing a role of transcription factor. In the early stage of tendon injury, accumulated cytokines, including tumor necrosis factor-α (TNF-α), interleukin-1β and -6 (ILs) act on the surface of tendon cells by Toll-like receptor, which activates NF-κB and then up regulates the expression of the above inflammatory factors to form positive feedback, amplifying inflammatory effect [81, 82]. Abraham et al. have found that inhibition of NF-κB signaling pathway by blocking I-kappaB kinase beta could mitigate tendinopathy development [83].

The TGF-β signaling pathway is widely studied in the pathological process of tendon adhesion formation. Smads proteins 2 and 3 (SMAD2/3) are molecules acting as a transcription factor of TGF-β as well as a signal transducer in the TGF-β pathway [84, 85]. The activated TGF-β acts on the fibroblasts and then phosphorylates the Smad2/3 protein in the cytoplasm to regulate the expression of target genes promoting fibroblasts proliferation and differentiation into myofibroblasts, so as to promote collagen secretion [86–89]. Down-regulate expression of TGF-β may significantly inhibit tendon adhesion formation. Wu el al. designed a three-dimensional tendon scaffold loading with *TGF-β* small interfering RNA (siRNA) plasmid and proved its satisfactory efficiency on prevention of tendon adhesion formation as well as promotion of tendon function repair [90]. Interestingly, after activated TGF-β binding to its receptor, extracellular signal-regulated kinase 1 and 2 (ERK1/2) which belongs to mitogen-activated protein kinases (MAPKs) pathways are also phosphorylated simultaneously to act on the binding sites of SMAD2/3, indirectly enhancing TGF-β/SMAD2/3 signaling pathway to promote exogenous fibroblast proliferation and collagen synthesis [86, 91, 92]. It indicated that the TGF-β signaling pathway could work in conjunction with other pathways like the MAPK pathway or BMP pathway [93].

Matrix metalloproteinase (MMP) is a protease family with metal ions as cofactors. TGF-β can induce the expression of plasminogen activator inhibitor-1 (PAL-1) in tenocytes to accelerate the degradation of plasmin and its mediated MMP-2, leading to excessive deposition of extracellular matrix (ECM) and type I collagen [94–96]. Lu et al. [97] confirmed that MMP comes from bone marrow cells that migrate to the injury site significantly enhance regeneration of tendon as well as tendon adhesion formation. Cai et al. [98] constructed a macrophage reactive siMMP hydrogel for high efficient synergistic prevention of tendon adhesion formation.

Besides, cyclooxygenase-2 (COX-2)/prostaglandin E (PGE)/prostaglandin type 4 receptor (EP4) signal transduction pathway also promote the tendon adhesion formation. It is found that the content of COX2 increases during tendon healing process, which can catalyze the decomposition of arachidonic acid into PGE acting on EP4 located in cell membrane to contribute to synthesis and accumulation of ECM [99–101]. Therefore, inhibition of COX2/PGE/EP4 signaling pathway may reduce the formation of tendon adhesion. However, some researches have demonstrated that the inhibition of COX-2 by high-dose utilization of non-steroidal anti-inflammatory drugs (NSAIDs) can increase the apoptosis of tenocytes recruited to defect sites, which is not conducive to tendon healing [102–104]. Furthermore, systemic application of EP4 inhibitor can increase the infiltration of macrophages and the secretion of type 1 collagen aggravating the degree of tendon adhesion [105]. In conclusion, the role of COX-2/PGE/EP4 signaling pathway in tendon adhesion formation is complex indicating more requirements for further studies on mechanism and more cautious usage of NSAIDs.

Altogether, it should be noted that tendon adhesion is a complex pathology process under the guidelines of multiple signaling pathways that interact with each other participating with various cytokines, growth factors and cells. Although studies on single regulation or recently synergistic regulation of signaling pathways have shown satisfactory outcomes in tendon adhesion prevention and tendon healing promotion, fully understanding on how exactly these signaling transduction pathways interact is on great demand.

2.3.5 Infections

Infection is mostly caused by a significant degree of contamination during the initial tendon injury [2, 7, 106]. The infection rate and severity depend on where the injury happens and how it is caused [107, 108]. And a review paper in 2018 reported the most common bacterial populations causing tendon adhesion formation even some devastating effects like gangrenosis. Therefore, it should be highly noted that infection which can mediate tendon adhesion formation should be completely forbidden, and recent study shows that it is capable to integrate an antimicrobial biomaterial. Shalumon et al. [109] constructed a multifunctional electrospun nanofiber membrane to perform excellent anti-infection effect as well as prolonged prevention of inflammation and tendon adhesion formation.

3. Tranditional strategies against tendon adhesion

Surgical intervention is usually unavoidable because lacerated tendon cannot repair by themselves and may retract and have remarkable defects after injury. Meanwhile, simultaneous injuries of adjacent skin, nerves, vessels, and bones also require surgical repair.

3.1 Intraoperative repair methods and tendon adhesion

Modified Kessler suture technique remains globally accepted method for flexor tendon repair with reliable mechanical strength and less peritendinous adhesion [3]. However, even if different modifications for tendon suture have been studied for decades, peritendinous adhesion often occurs and reoperation is still required due to undesired scar tissue formation [4, 110]. When it comes to tendon defect reconstruction, adhesion mechanism of autologous tenograft is believed to involve both intrinsic tenocyte necrosis and extrinsic fibrogenetic and inflammatory cell invasion, while mild peritendinous adhesion was observed in decellularized tendon allograft transplantation since the intrinsic mechanism was forbidden [106, 111]. Rather than adhesion formation, xenograft transplantation for tendon reconstruction may raise another important issue, high postoperative infection rate [112].

Physical barriers made of non-degradable materials including silica gel and gold foil have been previously applied intraoperatively to reduce peritendinous adhesion by wrapping the injured site [113]. However, these barriers are outdated and clinical application are eliminating since their non-degradability and non-permiability may prevent substance exchange and eventual tendon necrosis [24].

3.2 Pharmaceutic intervention

The use of anti-inflammatory drugs against tendon adhesion dates back to the 1980s when NSAIDs were simply injected to the injured area to reduce expression of pro-inflammatory factors that might promote scar tissue formation [114]. However, detrimental side effects of these drugs on cardiovascular and genitourinary systems sometimes occur when they are excessively used [115]. The effect of local steroid administration has been documented by several earlier studies as a dose-related decreased fibrogenesis, collagenesis, adhesion and tensile strength of the repaired tendon [116]. However, a recent animal study has also reported increased risk of peritendinous adhesion [117]. In the contrast, the controlled release of steroid by entrapping them with synthetic polymers showed promising antiadhesion and antiinflammatory effects in recent years [118]. To date, there is no consensus on whether steroid application should be a standard therapy for tendon adhesion.

4. Advanced materials against tendon adhesion

4.1 Basic characteristics

Taking advantage of advanced knowledge of materials, several polymeric or biogenetic materials have been studied and exploited as alternatives for conventional tendon restore strategies [12, 20, 119, 120]. Except for antiadhesion functionality, a few characteristics should be acquired for such materials, which include biodegradability, biocompatibility, accessibility with proper architecture, and reliable mechanical properties [21].

Polymer implantation materials are not supposed to permanently stay in human body, indicating that these synthetic materials should be biodegradable to avoid certain side effects, such as rejection reaction. The degradation should not interfere with the mechanical properties of the materials until safe gliding can be performed by the injured tendon, and the by-product should not be toxic and can be eventually eliminated by the human body [121]. The degradability of these polymers has been proven to be related with molar mass, crystallinity, and mechanical loading [122–124]. On the other hand, biogenetic materials against tendon adhesion, such as amnion, autograft membranes and allograft tendon sheath and pericardium, as well as their derivations, once show ability to replace natural tendon sheath, should otherwise tolerate biodegradation in order to perform as eternal sheath instead.

Biocompatibility is described as nontoxic, noncarcinogenic, nonthrombogenic, nonimmunogenic characteristics, and proper response to the host of implantation materials [125]. For acceptable biocompatibility of polymeric materials, in vitro cell seeding test should announce a cell viability over 70% [126]. The structural architecture of the implantation materials should manipulate the process of antiadhesion by allowing exchange of information and material, including growth factors, drugs, hormones and degradation by-products. Also, sufficient porosity is required in order to promote neovascularization [127–129]. Synthetic strategies determine not only the processability of the material but also the mechanical properties. Thus, it is of importance that the processing technique should be easy and cost-efficient for clinical application, and mechanical strength of the construct should be able to tolerate certain impact, e.g. tensile tests, to identify its biomechanical stability [130].

4.2 Synthetic materials against tendon adhesion

4.2.1 Hydrogel

Hydrogels represent a bunch of polymers crosslinking hydrophobic groups and hydrophilic residues with large water content, high porosity and similarity to extracellular environment. The hydrophobic outer layer stands for a physical barrier to isolate exogenous inflammatory response and inhibit fibroblast and macrophage migration during tendon repair, while the hydrophilic inner layer mimics the inner side of tendon sheath to direct and lubricate tendon gliding [131]. Topographic structure of hydrogel allows for carrying certain therapeutic agents to promote tendon healing and inhibit tendon adhesion. By controlling raw material concentration and crosslinking levels, appropriate hydrogel can be obtained with desired mechanical properties and degradation rate (**Figure 2**) [119, 131].

Hyaluronic acid (HA) is a kind of hydrophilic polysaccharide component of natural synovial fluid. With negative charge, its antiadhesion ability was confirmed by inhibiting fibroblast proliferation and migration [18]. Besides, HA exhibits an essential source of nutrition and lubrication for tendon gliding and repair, with strong potential in eliminating harmful inflammatory factors [132]. Hundreds of injectable hydrogel-based materials have been developed with the participation of HA in order to prevent peritendinous adhesion, among which Seprafilm, consisting of carboxymethylcellulose and HA, and xanthan gum/gellan gum/hyaluronan hydrogel showed both biocompatibility and antiadhesion efficacy *in vitro* and in *vivo* [133, 134].

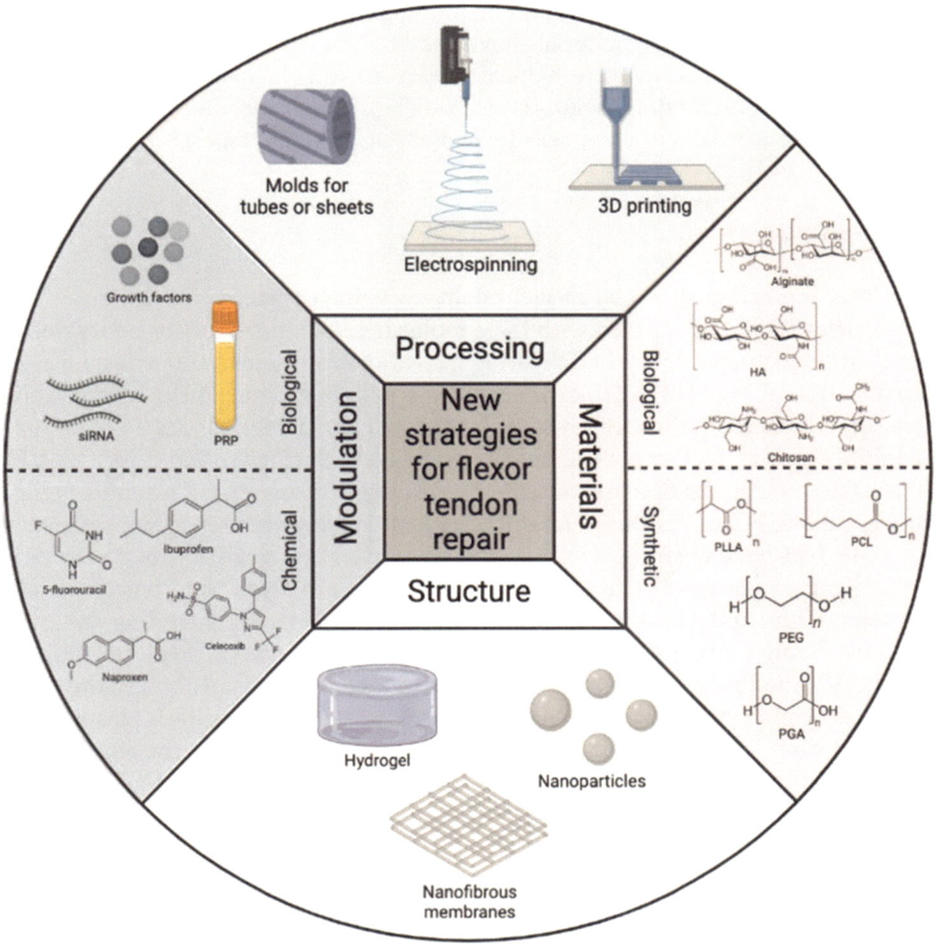

Figure 2.
Basic design considerations of therapeutic platforms for prevention of peritendinous adhesion including fabrication technologies, scaffold materials, therapeutic structures, and drug-loading.

Phospholipid-based hydrogels possess considerable biocompatibility in antiadhesion application as they do not induce foreign body reaction or cause protein conformational changes [135, 136]. Controllable degradation rate of such hydrogels can be achieved by altering the rate of coordinating compound [136]. Injectable hydrogels show great potential in inhibiting tendon adhesion because of its convenient, cost-effective, and minimally invasive manner in postsurgery rehabilitation, and the potential can be amplified when cross-linked with functional molecules. By integrating thermo-responsive material with chitosan and HA, liquid hydrogel will transfer to gel state and suit the tendon defect once body temperature is reached, and then chitosan plays its cytostatic role locally by suppressing fibroblast growth and infiltration [137, 138]. Solely applying chemosynthetic hydrogel remains less satisfactory due to nonspecific blocking adhesion as physical barrier. Therefore, developing drug-delivery platform with formulated hydrogel becomes an alternative method for inhibiting peritendinous adhesion. Cyclooxygenase-engineered miRNA plasmid-loaded polymer nanoparticles has been designed to be encapsulated into HA hydrogel to extend plasmid release against oxidative stress and adheasion formation during tendon repair [139]. Besides, appropriate 5-fluorouracil loading of hydrogel was proved to suppress fibroblast proliferation and migration. Despite the fact that these agent-hydrogel crosslinking materials have shown remarkable ability in the aspect of antiadhesion, a lack of proper mechanical properties still challenges their application in mimicking natural tendon sheath tissue, which promotes proliferation and tenogenic differentiation of stem cells by possessing suitable tensile loading and elasticity [17, 140].

4.2.2 Nanoparticles

Another important therapeutic agent delivery vehicle system is various nanoparticles (NPs). Compared with large molecules, NPs have shown better delivery efficacy and biocompatibility in delivering growth factors, genes and drugs by easier internalization of cells [141]. Quicker escaping from endosomes of the NPs also eliminates cargo biodegradation and thus prolongs bioactive cargo release [142].

Multiple growth factors have shown essential roles during tendon repair, as VEGF enhances neovascularization and accelerates healing process, PDGF promotes tendon gliding, and bFGF induces the differentiation of MSCs towards tenogenic linkage [143, 144]. NPs have been reported to serve as nonviral vectors for growth factors genes delivery, such as *bFGF* and *VEGF*, to induce overexpression in tenocytes of lacerated tendon, and downstream macromorphological effects, including enhanced tendon mechanical strength and tendon gliding, were observed *in vivo*, indicating satisfactory antiadhesion function of the transfected genes [66]. Although the NPs system has been proved to restrain adhesion by loading *TGF-β* miRNA plasmid for weeks, and simplify the procedure by minimally invasive injection, the absence of rigid mechanical strength of these particles forbids them from acting as physical barriers to separate ruptured tendon from surrounding tissue and migrating inflammatory cells [24]. Similar obstacle was also faced by antiadhesion nanoparticle-coated suture, as no proper timberland could separate the extrinsic healing and cell invasion [145]. New insights of employing self-healing HA hydrogel with NPs entrapping antiadhesion molecules may be reliable solutions to avoid unexpected artificial physical barrier rupture during tendon gliding. Cai et al. [98] reported successful inhibition of fibroblast proliferation and peritendinous adhesion in murine model with self-healing HA hydrogel loading *Smad3*-siRNA nanoparticles.

4.2.3 Nanofibrous membranes

Nanofibrous membranes (NFMs) have been approved as both reliable antiadhesion barriers and effective carriers of pharmaceutical agents due to their functional characteristics in the aspects of systematically and locally delivering medication, stem cells, components of ECM and genes, and being as physical goalkeepers inhibiting adhesion related to external tendon healing [127–129, 146, 147].

Among multiple methods to produce such NFMs, electrospinning remains one of the most popular ones for the fabrication of different nanofibers with diverse biomedical applications. Manufactured with this convenient and robust technique, the electrospun scaffolds share similar characteristics with natural ECM including topography and high porosity, and their mechanical properties can be easily modulated by altering the fiber alignment and diameter, and by manipulating the viscosity and volatility of the solution, applied voltage, flow rate of each polymer, along with the distance between the capillary and the collectors.

The electrospun NFMs should defend their payload against rapid degradation and permit release of the drugs or molecules in desired patterns for their antiadhesion applications. By controlling the material composition, drug-encapsulation technology and the architecture of the NFMs, this delivery system has been modified in order to optimizing its pharmacodynamics.

A variety of techniques, including surface modification, blending, coaxial and emulsion electrospinning, have been employed in order to encapsulate pharmaceutic agents into these nanofibers [148]. By physically and chemically altering the surface of the nanofibers with biomolecules, the surface modification technique is usually applied for vulnerable agents such as nucleic acids, proteins, growth factors and polysaccharides, which possess swift biodegradation rate and may lose their functionality during the process of electrospinning [149–154]. The rest three techniques were then established to accomplish gradual release of the therapeutic molecules. The blending technique requires the drugs or molecules to be dissolved in a polymeric solution before electrospinning, in which process the compatibility of the polymer and the solvend depends on the wettability to provide appropriate drug solubility and distribution [148, 150]. Coaxial electrospinning refers to the modification of traditional electrospinning process by concentrically locating the therapeutic cargoes during nanofiber fabrication, which will protect the biomolecules from environmental risks and attenuate drug degradation thus extending release period [155, 156]. Another effective method to prolong the drug release period is emulsion electrospinning, through which the organic solvent evaporates faster than the aqueous phase in which dissolves the molecular cargoes, leading to central migration of the biomolecules [157–160]. Besides, sequential electrospinning technique has been widely utilized to produce multi-layered NFMs which combine hydrophilicity or hydrophobia as well as mechanical strength and permeability of each layer of polymer, lubricate the tendons wrapped inside, and protect the longevity of the delivered molecules in order to release them during desired periods [161–164].

A wide spectrum of electrospun NFMs with diverse properties has been employed as flexible delivery platforms for pharmaceutic agents as well as nanoparticles to inhibit peritendinous adhesion. Despite alleviating tendon adhesion, the rapid clearance of NSAIDs and side effects on tendon repair limit their application for tendon healing and adhesion prevention. By loading ibuprofen (IBU) to poly (l-lactic acid)-polyethylene glycol (PELA) NFMs, Liu et al. [128] revealed that the delivery system could decrease peritendinous adhesion and kinetics of drug release was proved to be mostly dependent on its diffusion and polymer matrix degradation. Besides, more effective blocking of cell adhesion/proliferation and inflammation could be achieved by incorporating low content of polyethylene glycol (PEG) with PELA nanofibers [128]. To reduce postsurgical peritendinous adhesion with long-lasting release of NSAIDs, modified mesoporous silica (MMS) nanoparticles loading IBU was prepared and encapsulated within poly (l-lactic acid) (PLLA) nanofibers with emulsion electrospinning technique [165–167]. This IBU-MMS-PLLA drug delivery scaffold sustained release of drug by entrapping IBU within the porous MMS particles and its antiadhesion and antiinflammation functionality was observed even 8 weeks postoperatively. HA represents a widely used agent in preventing postsurgical adhesion and permitting tendon gliding due to its features of synovial fluid. By coating poly (ε-caprolactone) (PCL) with HA from the inner side, a bi-layer PCL/HA-PCL NFM has been reported to mimic tendon sheath as the outer layer PCL reduced cell adhesion/invasion and pro-inflammatory cytokine penetration, while the inner layer of HA lubricated the tendon and promoted gliding and healing [146]. Chitosan is another well-known polymer that can enhance the mechanical strength of NFMs when hybridized with other polymers, such as PCL, but the effect of chitosan-based NFMs against peritendinous adhesion remains controversial [147]. Although the hydrophilic nature of chitosan may partially reduce surface adhesion, other factors, including electric charge and roughness of the NFM also influences fibroblast attachment and recent studies have confirmed that PCL/chitosan NFMs had little impact on decreasing peritendinous adhesion [19, 168–171]. Meanwhile, the efficacy of loading certain particles to HA and then merging the HA-particle cargo to NFMs has also been well studied in terms of antiadhesion. Although mitomycin (MMC)-induced fibroblast apoptosis can inhibit collagen synthesis and is supposed to reduce tendon adhesion, misguided use of MMC may result in local and systematic toxicity [172]. By wrapping MMC in HA hydrogel and encapsulating the composite particle in PLLA nanofibers, notably controlled release of MMC was achieved and inhibition of tendon adhesion was observed *in vivo* [159]. Postsurgical infection also presents and important risk factor for peritendinous adhesion due to inflammation cascade and fibroblast infiltration [109]. Since silver (Ag) and its derived nanoparticles have shown strong antibacterial properties, NFMs with cored HA and Ag nanoparticles embedded in PCL shell have been investigated to possess adhesion prevention functionality [173]. Controlled release of the cored HA could promote tendon gliding and reduce fibroblast attachment, while the Ag nanoparticle-loaded NFM sheath with thinner diameter showed better capability of preventing fibroblast attachment *in vitro* and inhibiting peritendinous adhesion *in vivo* [174].

Incorporating biologics, including stem cells and growth factors, with NFMs scaffolds has recently gained significant attention in the field of tendon repair and antiadhesion [175]. Researchers have also attempted to load growth factors into nanofibers to exploit their antiinflammation and antiadhesion bioactivities, but the growth factors degrade easily when exposed to *in vivo* conditions and may be damaged during electrospinning preparation [65, 143]. Thus, similar to the afore-mentioned drug-nanoparticle-nanofiber delivery system, fabricating NFMs carrying growth factor-loaded nanoparticles may result in satisfying application of growth factors to prevent peritendinous adhesion. For instance, bFGF-loaded dextran glassy nanoparticles (DGNs) have been reported to contain higher proportion, less burst release and better-preserved bioactivity of bFGF when pre-formulated and encapsulated with PLLA nanofibers using the emulsion electrospinning technique, compared with bFGF-loaded PLLA, and in vivo investigations revealed that the bFGF-DGNs-

PLLA NFM scaffold not only promoted tendon healing but also mediated collagen remodeling in ECM and reduced tendon adhesion [176]. However, few attempts were taken to eliminate tendon adhesion by delivering stem cells with NFM scaffold. Liao et al. [177] found no significant reduction in tendon adhesion, despite the delivery of MSCs with minimal burst release using bi-layered HA/copolyermized l-lactide and ε-caprolactone NFMs, indicating a plenty of scope and opportunities for this approach.

Given the fact that inhibiting crucial cellular signaling pathways would reduce formation of adhesion, NFMs loading exogenous genetic materials have been developed to alter expression of certain genes related to peritendinous adhesion [178]. Small interfering RNA downregulating expression of ERK2 and SMAD2/3 has been shown to prevent fibroblast proliferation as well as abnormal collagen accumulation [179]. To employ such functionality, a pyridinedicarboxaldehyde-polyethylenimine (PDA)-mediated exogenous *ERK2*-siRNA delivery system based on PLLA/hyaluronan (P/H) nanofiber scaffold has been developed in order to gradually inhibit ERK2 bioactivity and reduce peritendinous adhesion [178]. *In vivo* model demonstrated that *ERK2*-siRNA-PDA-P/H delivery system could reduce type III collagen density through down-regulating *ERK2* and *SMAD3* gene expression, thus inhibiting tendon adhesion (**Table 1**).

4.3 Biomimetic materials against tendon adhesion

4.3.1 Amnion and its deviations

Human amniotic membrane (HAM) tissue is inexpensive, easily stored, of minimal antigenicity and with low immunogenic rejection, and has shown advanced potential in preventing postsurgical adhesion [186]. Recent findings also revealed its reinforcement on mechanical strength after combined with modified Kessler suture in flexor tendon repair, probably due to the expression of multiple growth factors that promotes tenocyte proliferation [187, 188]. The decellularized HAM can physically inhibit cell infiltration and preserve tendon gliding through "tunnel effect", and biochemically suppress ILs-induced immunologic cascade to alleviate systematic inflammatory response and local abnormal collagen synthesis [189–193].

Typical strategy to apply HAM and other films to the injured site of tendon generally depends on wrapping and suture. However, excessive suture burden may also result in consequent fibrogenesis and adhesion, stimulated by the suture as foreign body. To reduce such complications, several modification techniques has been employed for HAM modification. Photochemical tissue bonding (PTB) technique requires photo-active substance, e.g. Rose Bengal (RB), to conglutinate tissues through illumination [194]. Ding et al. [27] found that by immersing decellularized HAM in 0.1% (w/v) RB, attaching HAM to repaired chicken tendon became sutureless and significantly reduced inflammatory cell chemotaxis and better joint performance were observed. Wrapping freeze-dried HAM around the sutured site of lacerated tendon may also result in moderate peritendinous adhesion because of the uncontrolled expression and emission of TGF-β, which promotes exogenous fibroblast migration and collagen synthesis through ERK/SMAD pathway [24]. Coating PCL on both surfaces of the HAM by electrospinning technique has been identified in a rabbit model to reduce such adhesion by (1) prevent outer fibroblast and inflammatory infiltration, (2) gradual release of multiple growth factors, e.g. PDGF, VEGF, and TGF-β from the intermediate HAM layer, and (3) maintaining tendon gliding inside the membrane, thanks to the appropriate porous network of the PCL NFMs [195].

Researchers	Type of material	Source of material	Molecule loading	Manufacture	Mechanical strength	Cell line	*In vitro* results	Animal model	*In vivo* results	Publication year	Publication title
Liu et al.	biomimetic bilayer sheath membrane	PCL, HA	HA	combination of sequential and microgel electrospinning technologies	bilayer of PCL-HA0%:2.13 ± 0.25 MPa PCL-HA4%:1.91 ± 0.21 MPa PCLHA8%:1.77 ± 0.18 MPa PCL-HA12%:1.55 ± 0.21 MPa	multipotent C3H10T1/2cells	More cells adhered to and were better distributed on the surface of the inner HA-loaded PCL layer and the tissue culture plate surfaces	flexor tendon of Leghorn chickens	The average scores of adhesions and tendon healing in the biomimetic bilayer sheath membrane group were lower than the other groups	2012	Biomimetic sheath membrane via electrospinning for antiadhesion of the repaired tendon
Liu et al.	Electrospun fibrous membranes	PELA	Ibuprofen	electrospinning	Maximum tensile strength (MPa) PELA-0% 3.72 ± 0.32, PELA-2% 3.42 ± 0.36, PELA-6% 3.13 ± 0.38, PELA-10% 2.89 ± 0.31	L929 mouse fibroblast	Fewer cells adhered to the ibuprofen-loaded PELA fibers	flexor digitorum profundus tendons of Leghorn chickens	No peritendinous adhesions were detected in most tendons treated with the ibuprofen-loaded PELA fibrous membrane	2013	Prevention of Peritendinous Adhesions with Electrospun Ibuprofen-Loaded Poly(L-Lactic Acid)-Polyethylene Glycol Fibrous Membranes
Liu et al.	Electrospun fibrous membranes	PLLA	dextran glassy nanoparticles (DGNs) loaded with bFGF	electrospinning	Tensile strength(MPA) PLLA 4.38 ± 0.33, bFGF PLLA 4.38 ± 0.33 and bFGF/DGNs-PLLA fibrous membranes 3.54 ± 0.25	multipotent C3H10T½ (C3) cells	The PLLA membrane showed an anti-adhesion effect, more cells adhered to and were better distributed on the surface of the bFGF/DGNs-PLLA membrane	Achilles tendon of male SD rats	In the bFGF/DGNs-PLLA group, A significantly increased tendon thickness was observed, tendon healing and vascular prominence and angiogenesis were significantly better, and an increase in breaking force	2013	Tendon healing and anti-adhesion properties of electrospun fibrous membranes containing bFGF loaded nanoparticles

Researchers	Type of material	Source of material	Molecule loading	Manufacture	Mechanical strength	Cell line	*In vitro* results	Animal model	*In vivo* results	Publication year	Publication title
									was detected but still lower than control group.		
Kuo et al.	Hydrogel	xanthan gum/gellan gum/ hyaluronan hydrogel	/	Blending	/	/	/	Achilles tendon of SD rats	Help reduce the incidence of postoperative tendon adhesion, and enable tendon healing and preserve the mechanical strength as effectively as Seprafilm.	2014	Evaluation of the ability of xanthan gum gellan gum hyaluronan hydrogel membranes to prevent the adhesion of postrepaired tendons
Chen et al.	nanofibrous membrane	chitosan-grafted PCL	/	electrospinning	Ultimate tensile strength (MPa) PCL1.4 ± 0.1, PCL-g-CS 2.2 ± 0.5	Human foreskin fibroblast (Hs68) cells	The inhibition of cell migration by PCL-g-CS NFMs was evident, and the CS layer on the PCL-g-CS NFM can prevent more nonspecific cell adhesion.	flexor digitorum profundus of New Zealand white rabbits	In the tendons treated with the PCL-g-CS NFM, no adhesion was observed, There was a statistical improvement in the DIP joint flexion angle, PIP joint flexion angle and sliding excursion. And tendons treated with PCL-g-CS NFM required the least pull-out force and showed the lowest degree of stiffness.	2014	Prevention of peritendinous adhesions with electrospun chitosan-grafted polycaprolactone nanofibrous membranes

Researchers	Type of material	Source of material	Molecule loading	Manufacture	Mechanical strength	Cell line	*In vitro* results	Animal model	*In vivo* results	Publication year	Publication title
Chen et al.	nanofibrous membrane	HA, PCL, PEO	Ag	electrospinning		human foreskin fibroblasts (Hs68)	Compared to other NFMs, the lowest number of cells and the least cell spreading were found on the PCL/HA + Ag NFMs.	flexor tendon of New Zealand white rabbits	The surface of the repaired tendon was smooth, and no adhesion was observed between the repaired tendon and the peritendinous tissue. No adhesions were observed between the repaired tendon and the surrounding tissue in the HA/PCL + Ag NFM treatment group	2015	Dual functional core-sheath electrospun hyaluronic acid/ polycaprolactone nanofibrous membranes embedded with silver nanoparticles for prevention of peritendinous adhesion
Tang et al.	Nanoparticle	PEI-modified PLGA	AAV2-TGF-β1-miRNA	solvent evaporation	/	Rabbit tenocytes	significantly improved the expression of the gene of type I collagen	flexor digitorum profundus tendons of chickens	Gene therapy through AAV2 vectors is efficient to deliver growth factor genes to the healing tendon and reduce adhesion formations, but reduces in tendon healing strength	2016	Gene therapy strategies to improve strength and quality of flexor tendon healing

Researchers	Type of material	Source of material	Molecule loading	Manufacture	Mechanical strength	Cell line	*In vitro* results	Animal model	*In vivo* results	Publication year	Publication title
Liu et al.	Electrospun nanofibers menbrane	PLA	Ibuprofen	Blending	/	RAW264.7 macrophages	Less RAW264.7 adhered to the surface of IBU/PLA-M than to the surface of PLA-M.	flexor digitorum profundus tendons of Leghorn chickens	Although granuloma formation was investigated in the IBU/PLA-M group, a clear space around the tendon could usually be observed. The number of α-SMA positive vessels in the IBU/PLA-M group is significantly lower than that in the PLA-M group.	2017	Macrophage infiltration of electrospun polyester fibers
Zhou et al.	Hydrogel	thiol-modified hyaluronic acid/PEG-diacrylate	COX-1 and COX-2 miRNA plasmids	Blending	The elastic modulus, yield strength, and elongation to yield for hydrogel are 0.121 ± 0.01 MPa, 0.014 ± 0.003 MPa, and 3.50% ± 0.5%, respectively.			flexor digitorum profundus tendons of white Leghorn chickens	This hydrogel could effectively reduce the expression of COX-1 and COX-2 proteins in the tendons and subcutaneous tissues.	2018	Localized delivery of miRNAs targets cyclooxygenases and reduces flexor tendon adhesions
Chen et al.	Micro-hydrogel-generated asymmetric scaffold	chitosan	tendon stem/progenitor cells	Self-deposition technique	641.61 ± 12.43 MPa	tendon stem/progenitor cells sided onto the scaffold	displayed higher levels of tenogenic specific genes expression and protein production.	Achilles tendon of SD rats	synergistic effect on tendon regeneration and yielded better-aligned collagen fibers with elongated, spindle-shaped cells.	2018	An asymmetric chitosan scaffold for tendon tissue engineering

Researchers	Type of material	Source of material	Molecule loading	Manufacture	Mechanical strength	Cell line	*In vitro* results	Animal model	*In vivo* results	Publication year	Publication title
Jayasree et al	Electrospun menbrane	PCL-Collagen-bFGF	PCL, collagen bFGF nanofiber	electrospinning	89.4 ± 5.3 MPa	Rabbit tenocyte	Upon dynamic stimulation, mPCL-nCol-bFGF-DS scaffolds showed significantly higher expression of tenascin C, collagen I, biglycan, and fibronectin.	Achilles tendon of New Zealand white rabbits	The alignment of collagen was highly in comparison to native tendon which showed perfectly aligned fiber morphology, whereas, by 12 weeks, the implants showed more aligned nature of collagen fibers which was further confirmed by MT staining.	2019	Bioengineered Braided Micro-Nano (Multiscale) Fibrous Scaffolds for Tendon Reconstruction
Park et al.	film	cross-linked electrospun cartilage acellular matrix (CAM)	CAM, PLGA	cross-linking	25.06 ± 1.4 N	L929 mouse fibroblast cells	Cell migration from serum-free medium area towards serum containing medium area was inhibited in the CX-CAM film group	Achilles tendon of New Zealand White rabbits	The degree of adhesion in histology was highest in the repair group, followed by Seprafilm, CX-CAM film, and sham group.	2020	Cross-linked cartilage acellular matrix film decreases postsurgical peritendinous adhesions
Song et al.	Electrospun menbrane	PCL	mechano-growth factor	Electrospinning	/	RAW264.7 mouse macrophages	Antiinflammatory macrophage phenotype polarization	Achilles tendon of SD rats	Almost no adhesion can be detected in the MGF-modified group with a sheath space formed between tendon and scaffold.	2021	Surface modification of electrospun fibers with mechano-growth factor for mitigating the foreign-body reaction

DOI: http://dx.doi.org/10.5772/intechopen.108019

Researchers	Type of material	Source of material	Molecule loading	Manufacture	Mechanical strength	Cell line	*In vitro* results	Animal model	*In vivo* results	Publication year	Publication title
Chen et al.	Core-sheath nanofiber membrane	PLA, HA,	Ag/Tn/Tk	Blending and core-shell	/	NIH/3 T3 mouse embryonic fibroblasts	A synergistic effect was found by combining Ag NPs with HA as Tn+, with Ag NPs embedded in the thin sheath and the highest amount of released HA, which demonstrated the least staining of vinculin by inhibiting cell adhesion as well as suppressing cell spreading.	flexor digitorum profundus tendons of New Zealand White rabbits	The Tn + group showed a nearly complete lack of adhesion and demonstrated the most regular collagen arrangement.	2021	Functional Hyaluronic Acid-Polylactic Acid/ Silver Nanoparticles Core-Sheath Nanofiber Membranes for Prevention of PostOperative Tendon Adhesion

Source: [128, 139, 146, 173, 174, 176, 180–185]

Table 1.
Recent research on biomaterials for the prevention of peritendinous adhesion.

HAM and its deviations have been gradually utilized in preventing peritendinous adhesion during clinical practice. Compared with synthesized polymer membrane and control group, HAM has been reported to significantly attenuated complication rate of erythema, exudate and rupture in repaired Zone II human flexor tendons, but there was no difference in ultimate interphalangeal joint range of motion [196]. In addition, local administration of HAM wrapping around injured human flexor tendon was observed to reduce serum level of IL-6 and TGF-β1, indicating a systematic antiinflammation effect during tendon repair, thus preventing tendon adhesion [190]. On the other hand, effect of HAM allograft against tendon adhesion, tenolysis and joint complications after application in flexor tendon repair was questioned by Leppänen et al. [197] since half of the 10 patients enrolled developed these complications.

4.3.2 Tendon and sheath graft and reconstruction

Two-stage flexor tendon defect reconstruction remains gold standard [198]. The technique requires first-stage silicone rod insertion for tendon pseudo-sheath formation for at least 3 months and second-stage rod removal with tendon grafting. Functional results of this technique are not always predictable, which also depend a lot on patient's compliance with prolonged duration of rehabilitation and time off work [106]. By employing tubular polyurethane nanocomposite graft surrounding autologous tenograft, single-staged flexor tendon reconstruction in sheep hind extremity model revealed mild histological adhesion and satisfactory tendon gliding [199]. In addition to artificial synovial graft, the *in vivo* experimental study of artificial tendon substitution assembled with platelet gel-collagen-polydioxanone has also shed light on promising Achilles tendon healing and adhesion prevention [26, 200]. It is believed that abundant PDGF level in such platelet gel may alter fibro-adiogenic progenitors from fibrotic differentiation towards tendon stem cells, thus relatively alleviate scar tissue formation [201].

Two-stage extensor tendon reconstruction is not a preferable approach in reported literature because of the absence of fibroosseous sheath guiding both extrinsic and intrinsic musculotendinous movement [202]. However, one-stage extensor tendon reconstruction may be accompanied with subsequent adhesion in cases with multiple soft tissue defect, severe contamination, and bone defect or fracture which requires long-term immobilization [203, 204]. In those cases, first-stage artificial tendon substitutions insertion, including silicone rods, can be an alternative method to maintain tendon route and form pseudo-synovial tunnel, to inhibit inflammation and infection, and thus to prevent adhesion formation for second-stage tendon grafting [205]. The use of such synthetic silicone rods has declined over years due to many complications, such as pyogenic tenosynovitis and high failure rate [206, 207].

Extra synovial tendon autografts are currently wide-accepted donor for tendon defect reconstruction. These tendons, such as palmaris longus, however, lack natural synovial cells mounted on loose connective tissue in tendons possessing sheaths, such as flexor digitorum superficialis. It has been observed in canine model that extra synovial tendon autograft underwent quicker cell death and ECM remodeling, and more excessive peritendinous adhesion, compared with intra synovial tendon autograft [208]. Explanation for such differences may lie in the different initial expression spectrum of these two kinds of tendons, and in their different response to the extracellular environment of the recipient site [209]. Rabbit model revealed that after 28 days of autograft transplantation using extra or intrasynovial tendon, donor segment showed different proteomic features in the expression of certain proteins, including heat shock protein 47, tenascin, periostin, etc., indicating the relationship among environmental stimuli around recipient site, oxidative stress, cell homeostasis and consequent peritendinous adhesion [23].

The availability of tendon allograft offers reconstruction options for patients without adequate tendon autograft reservation. Early studies have demonstrated triumphs in clinical flexor tendon reconstruction using fresh tendon allograft with composite sheath and volar plates, which, however, arouse concerns, including the harvesting and storing technique, transmission of diseases, and ethical issues [210]. Since programmed sterilization, decellularization and lyophilization have been shown to have little influence on biomechanical properties of composite tendon allograft, diverse modifications of such allograft have been studied to minimize postsurgery peritendinous adhesion [211, 212]. These modifications include synthetic polymer loading, tonogenic stem cell repopulation, and antiadhesion genes delivery, all of which were shown to reduce tendon graft gliding resistance in animal models [213–215]. Although safe and effective clinical use of lyophilized and sterilized tendon allograft has been reported in upper extremity reconstruction, no biologically modified acellular tendon allograft has been implanted in humans to date in the aim of preventing tenograft adhesion [216].

4.3.3 Pericardium as tendon sheath substitution

Due to the difficulties in tendon sheath suture with conventional surgical techniques, tendon sheath engineering has drawn wide attention in order to support tendon gliding and prevent peritendinous adhesion, apart from chemosynthetic materials. Typical biogenetic tendon sheath usually requires a scaffold, either from decellularized membraneous allograft or xenograft, or simple scaffold synthesized with collagen or lipoprotein, and techniques reseeding certain cells onto the membraneous scaffold. Bioengineered tendon sheath with collagen scaffold and harvested synoviocyte has been reported to inhibit Achilles tendon adhesion formation in rabbit model [217]. Porcine pericardium has also been applied as bioengineered tendon sheath scaffold since the pericardium functions similar as tendon sheath to lubricate heart beating, based on which decellularized bovine pericardium tendon xenograft and allograft have achieved successful adhesion prevention outcomes in chicken and donkey models [22]. Although Megerle et al. [25] did not test the tendon gliding resistance *in vivo*, their repopulationed human synoviocyte and adipose-derived stem cell on decellularized porcine pericardium showed shifted expression of downregulated collagen and upregulated hyaluronan synthase, suggesting potential antiadhesion mechanism during human cell line transplantation [218].

5. Conclusion

Taken together, the successful exploration and application of advanced antiadhesion materials highly depend on the collaboration among experts with diverse backgrounds, including engineering, biology, chemistry, surgeons, and sociologists. Intensive understanding of the pathophysiological procedure of tendon adhesion in combination with advanced material fabrication technologies will do a great favor to establishing next-generation of therapeutic platforms against tendon adhesion.

Author details

Shen Liu[1,2*], Qinglin Kang[1], Rui Zhang[1], Yanhao Li[1,2] and Rong Bao[1,2]

1 Department of Orthopaedics, Shanghai Sixth People's Hospital Affiliated to Shanghai Jiao Tong University School of Medicine, Shanghai, China

2 Shanghai Engineering Research Center for Orthopaedic Material Innovation and Tissue Regeneration, Shanghai, China

*Address all correspondence to: liushensjtu@126.com

References

[1] Apostolakos J et al. The enthesis: A review of the tendon-to-bone insertion. Muscle, Ligaments and Tendons Journal. 2014;**4**:333-342

[2] Millar NL et al. Tendinopathy. Nature Reviews Disease Primers. 2021;7:1

[3] Dy CJ et al. Complications after flexor tendon repair: A systematic review and meta-analysis. The Journal of Hand Surgery. 2012;**37**:543-551.e541

[4] Yoneda S et al. The effect of modified locking methods and suture materials on zone II flexor tendon repair-an ex vivo study. PLoS One. 2018;**13**:e0205121

[5] Titan AL, Foster DS, Chang J, Longaker MT. Flexor tendon: Development, healing, adhesion formation, and contributing growth factors. Plastic and Reconstructive Surgery. 2019;**144**:639e-647e

[6] Gelberman RH, Steinberg D, Amiel D, Akeson W. Fibroblast chemotaxis after tendon repair. The Journal of Hand Surgery. 1991;**16**: 686-693

[7] Pearce O, Brown MT, Fraser K, Lancerotto L. Flexor tendon injuries: Repair & Rehabilitation. Injury. 2021;**52**: 2053-2067

[8] Thomopoulos S, Parks WC, Rifkin DB, Derwin KA. Mechanisms of tendon injury and repair. Journal of Orthopaedic Research. 2015;**33**:832-839

[9] Taylor SH et al. Tendon is covered by a basement membrane epithelium that is required for cell retention and the prevention of adhesion formation. PLoS One. 2011;**6**:e16337

[10] Meier Burgisser G et al. Rabbit Achilles tendon full transection model—Wound healing, adhesion formation and biomechanics at 3, 6 and 12 weeks post-surgery. Biology Open. 2016;**5**: 1324-1333

[11] Liu CF et al. What we should know before using tissue engineering techniques to repair injured tendons: A developmental biology perspective. Tissue Engineering Reviews (Part B). 2011;**17**:165-176

[12] Zhou H, Lu H. Advances in the development of anti-adhesive biomaterials for tendon repair treatment. Tissue Engineering and Regenerative Medicine. 2021;**18**:1-14

[13] Schnuriger B et al. Prevention of postoperative peritoneal adhesions: A review of the literature. American Journal of Surgery. 2011;**201**:111-121

[14] Wu Y, Han Y, Wong YS, Fuh JYH. Fibre-based scaffolding techniques for tendon tissue engineering. Journal of Tissue Engineering and Regenerative Medicine. 2018;**12**:1798-1821

[15] Rademakers T, Horvath JM, van Blitterswijk CA, LaPointe VLS. Oxygen and nutrient delivery in tissue engineering: Approaches to graft vascularization. Journal of Tissue Engineering and Regenerative Medicine. 2019;**13**:1815-1829

[16] Cravedi P et al. Regenerative immunology: The immunological reaction to biomaterials. Transplant International. 2017;**30**:1199-1208

[17] No YJ, Castilho M, Ramaswamy Y, Zreiqat H. Role of biomaterials and controlled architecture on tendon/ ligament repair and regeneration. Advanced Materials. 2020;**32**:e1904511

[18] Thomas SC, Jones LC, Hungerford DS. Hyaluronic acid and its effect on postoperative adhesions in the rabbit flexor tendon. A preliminary look. Clinical Orthopaedics and Related Research. 1986;**206**:281-289

[19] Gomes SR et al. In vitro and in vivo evaluation of electrospun nanofibers of PCL, chitosan and gelatin: A comparative study. Materials Science & Engineering. C, Materials for Biological Applications. 2015;**46**:348-358

[20] Zhang Q et al. Advanced technology-driven therapeutic interventions for prevention of tendon adhesion: Design, intrinsic and extrinsic factor considerations. Acta Biomaterialia. 2021;**124**:15-32

[21] Brebels J, Mignon A. Polymer-based constructs for flexor tendon repair: A review. Polymers (Basel). 2022;**14**:867

[22] El-Shafaey ESA, Karrouf GI, Zaghloul AE. Clinical and biomechanical evaluation of three bioscaffold augmentation devices used for superficial digital flexor tenorrhaphy in donkeys (*Equus asinus*): An experimental study. Journal of Advanced Research. 2013;**4**:103-113

[23] Farnebo S, Wiig M, Holm B, Ghafouri B. Differentially expressed proteins in intra synovial compared to extra synovial flexor tendon grafts in a rabbit tendon transplantation model. Biomedicine. 2020;**8**:408

[24] Sang R et al. Effect of acellular amnion with increased TGF-beta and bFGF levels on the biological behavior of tenocytes. Frontiers in Bioengineering and Biotechnology. 2020;**8**:446

[25] Megerle K et al. Flexor tendon sheath engineering using decellularized porcine pericardium. Plastic and Reconstructive Surgery. 2016;**138**:630e-641e

[26] Oryan A, Moshiri A, Meimandi-Parizi A. Implantation of a novel tissue-engineered graft in a large tendon defect initiated inflammation, accelerated fibroplasia and improved remodeling of the new Achilles tendon: A comprehensive detailed study with new insights. Cell and Tissue Research. 2014; **355**:59-80

[27] Ding B, Wang X, Yao M. Photochemical tissue bonding technique for improving healing of hand tendon injury. Surgical Innovation. 2019;**26**: 153-161

[28] Kjaer M. Role of extracellular matrix in adaptation of tendon and skeletal muscle to mechanical loading. Physiological Reviews. 2004;**84**:649-698

[29] Kjaer M et al. From mechanical loading to collagen synthesis, structural changes and function in human tendon. Scandinavian Journal of Medicine & Science in Sports. 2009;**19**:500-510

[30] Birch HL. Tendon matrix composition and turnover in relation to functional requirements. International Journal of Experimental Pathology. 2007;**88**:241-248

[31] Ackermann PW, Hart DA. Metabolic influences on risk for tendon disorders preface. Advances in Experimental Medicine and Biology. 2016;**920**:V-Vi

[32] Thorpe CT, Screen HR. Tendon structure and composition. Advances in Experimental Medicine and Biology. 2016;**920**:3-10

[33] Barnard K, Light ND, Sims TJ, Bailey AJ. Chemistry of the collagen cross-links. Origin and partial characterization of a putative mature

cross-link of collagen. The Biochemical Journal. 1987;**244**:303-309

[34] Canty EG, Kadler KE. Procollagen trafficking, processing and fibrillogenesis. Journal of Cell Science. 2005;**118**:1341-1353

[35] Juncosa-Melvin N et al. Effects of mechanical stimulation on the biomechanics and histology of stem cell-collagen sponge constructs for rabbit patellar tendon repair. Tissue Engineering. 2006;**12**: 2291-2300

[36] Strickland JW. Development of flexor tendon surgery: Twenty-five years of progress. The Journal of Hand Surgery. 2000;**25**:214-235

[37] Lin TW, Cardenas L, Soslowsky LJ. Biomechanics of tendon injury and repair. Journal of Biomechanics. 2004;**37**: 865-877

[38] Nichols AEC, Best KT, Loiselle AE. The cellular basis of fibrotic tendon healing: Challenges and opportunities. Translational Research. 2019;**209**: 156-168

[39] Millar NL, Murrell GA, McInnes IB. Inflammatory mechanisms in tendinopathy—Towards translation. Nature Reviews Rheumatology. 2017;**13**: 110-122

[40] Manning CN et al. Adipose-derived mesenchymal stromal cells modulate tendon fibroblast responses to macrophage-induced inflammation in vitro. Stem Cell Research & Therapy. 2015;**6**:74

[41] Shen H et al. The effect of mesenchymal stromal cell sheets on the inflammatory stage of flexor tendon healing. Stem Cell Research & Therapy. 2016;**7**:144

[42] Koob TJ, Summers AP. Tendon–bridging the gap. Comparative Biochemistry and Physiology. Part A, Molecular & Integrative Physiology. 2002;**133**:905-909

[43] Strickland JW. Flexor tendons: Acute injuries. In: *Green's Operative Hand Surgery*. London, UK: Churchill Livingstone; 1999

[44] Das A et al. Monocyte and macrophage plasticity in tissue repair and regeneration. The American Journal of Pathology. 2015;**185**:2596-2606

[45] Wojciak B, Crossan JF. The accumulation of inflammatory cells in synovial sheath and epitenon during adhesion formation in healing rat flexor tendons. Clinical and Experimental Immunology. 1993;**93**:108-114

[46] Berglund ME et al. Neuropeptide, mast cell, and myofibroblast expression after rabbit deep flexor tendon repair. The Journal of Hand Surgery. 2010;**35**: 1842-1849

[47] Best KT, Loiselle AE. Scleraxis lineage cells contribute to organized bridging tissue during tendon healing and identify a subpopulation of resident tendon cells. The FASEB Journal. 2019; **33**:8578-8587

[48] Bi Y et al. Identification of tendon stem/progenitor cells and the role of the extracellular matrix in their niche. Nature Medicine. 2007;**13**:1219-1227

[49] Dyment NA et al. Lineage tracing of resident tendon progenitor cells during growth and natural healing. PLoS One. 2014;**9**:e96113

[50] Yoshida R et al. Murine supraspinatus tendon injury model to identify the cellular origins of rotator

cuff healing. Connective Tissue Research. 2016;**57**:507-515

[51] Tempfer H et al. Perivascular cells of the supraspinatus tendon express both tendon- and stem cell-related markers. Histochemistry and Cell Biology. 2009; **131**:733-741

[52] Mienaltowski MJ, Adams SM, Birk DE. Regional differences in stem cell/progenitor cell populations from the mouse achilles tendon. Tissue Engineering. Part A. 2013;**19**: 199-210

[53] Yin Z et al. Single-cell analysis reveals a nestin(+) tendon stem/ progenitor cell population with strong tenogenic potentiality. Science Advances. 2016;**2**:e1600874

[54] Sakabe T et al. Transcription factor scleraxis vitally contributes to progenitor lineage direction in wound healing of adult tendon in mice. The Journal of Biological Chemistry. 2018;**293**:5766-5780

[55] Darby IA, Laverdet B, Bonte F, Desmouliere A. Fibroblasts and myofibroblasts in wound healing. Clinical, Cosmetic and Investigational Dermatology. 2014;**7**:301-311

[56] Hu B, Phan SH. Myofibroblasts. Current Opinion in Rheumatology. 2013; **25**:71-77

[57] Docheva D, Muller SA, Majewski M, Evans CH. Biologics for tendon repair. Advanced Drug Delivery Reviews. 2015; **84**:222-239

[58] Branford OA, Klass BR, Grobbelaar AO, Rolfe KJ. The growth factors involved in flexor tendon repair and adhesion formation. The Journal of Hand Surgery (European Volume). 2014;**39**:60-70

[59] Voleti PB, Buckley MR, Soslowsky LJ. Tendon healing: Repair and regeneration. Annual Review of Biomedical Engineering. 2012;**14**:47-71

[60] Galvez MG, Crowe C, Farnebo S, Chang J. Tissue engineering in flexor tendon surgery: Current state and future advances. The Journal of Hand Surgery (European Volume). 2014;**39**:71-78

[61] Wu YF et al. Adeno-associated virus-2-mediated TGF-beta1 microRNA transfection inhibits adhesion formation after digital flexor tendon injury. Gene Therapy. 2016;**23**:167-175

[62] Lu H et al. Tanshinone IIA prevent tendon adhesion in the rat Achilles tendon model. Journal of Biomaterials and Tissue Engineering. 2016;**6**:739-744

[63] Tang JB et al. Basic FGF or VEGF gene therapy corrects insufficiency in the intrinsic healing capacity of tendons. Scientific Reports. 2016;**6**:20643

[64] Pan Q et al. Exosomes derived from mesenchymal stem cells ameliorate hypoxia/reoxygenation-injured ECs via transferring microRNA-126. Stem Cells International. **2019;2019**:2831756

[65] Evrova O, Buschmann J. In vitro and in vivo effects of Pdgf-bb delivery strategies on tendon healing: A review. European Cells & Materials. 2017;**34**: 15-39

[66] Yang QQ, Shao YX, Zhang LZ, Zhou YL. Therapeutic strategies for flexor tendon healing by nanoparticle-mediated co-delivery of bFGF and VEGFA genes. Colloids and Surfaces. B, Biointerfaces. 2018;**164**:165-176

[67] Shen H et al. BMP12 induces tenogenic differentiation of adipose-

derived stromal cells. PLoS One. 2013;**8**: e77613

[68] Wang D et al. BMP14 induces tenogenic differentiation of bone marrow mesenchymal stem cells in vitro. Experimental and Therapeutic Medicine. 2018;**16**:1165-1174

[69] Hyun SY, Lee JH, Kang KJ, Jang YJ. Effect of FGF-2, TGF-beta-1, and BMPs on Teno/Ligamentogenesis and osteo/ Cementogenesis of human periodontal ligament stem cells. Molecules and Cells. 2017;**40**:550-557

[70] de Aro AA et al. Injured Achilles tendons treated with adipose-derived stem cells transplantation and GDF-5. Cell. 2018;**7**:127

[71] Niu X et al. Tendon cell regeneration is mediated by attachment site-resident progenitors and BMP Signaling. Current Biology. 2020;**30**:3277-3292 e3275

[72] Chen S et al. Tenogenic adipose-derived stem cell sheets with nanoyarn scaffolds for tendon regeneration. Materials Science & Engineering. C, Materials for Biological Applications. 2021;**119**:111506

[73] Sarikaya B, Gumusderelioglu M. Aligned silk fibroin/poly-3-hydroxybutyrate nanofibrous scaffolds seeded with adipose-derived stem cells for tendon tissue engineering. International Journal of Biological Macromolecules. 2021;**193**:276-286

[74] Logerstedt DS et al. Effects of and response to mechanical loading on the knee. Sports Medicine. 2022;**52**:201-235

[75] Rinoldi C et al. Tendon tissue engineering: Effects of mechanical and biochemical stimulation on stem cell alignment on cell-laden hydrogel yarns. Advanced Healthcare Materials. 2019;**8**: e1801218

[76] Abdulmalik S et al. The glucagon-like peptide 1 receptor agonist Exendin-4 induces tenogenesis in human mesenchymal stem cells. Differentiation. 2021;**120**:1-9

[77] Olesen JL et al. No treatment benefits of local administration of insulin-like growth factor-1 in addition to heavy slow resistance training in tendinopathic human patellar tendons a randomized, double-blind, placebo-controlled trial with 1-year follow-up. The American Journal of Sports Medicine. 2021;**49**: 2361-2370

[78] Farnebo S et al. Optimized repopulation of tendon hydrogel: Synergistic effects of growth factor combinations and adipose-derived stem cells. Hand (New York, N.Y.). 2017;**12**: 68-77

[79] Holladay C et al. Preferential tendon stem cell response to growth factor supplementation. Journal of Tissue Engineering and Regenerative Medicine. 2016;**10**:783-798

[80] Chan KM et al. Expression of transforming growth factor beta isoforms and their roles in tendon healing. Wound Repair and Regeneration. 2008;**16**:399-407

[81] Hoesel B, Schmid JA. The complexity of NF-kappa B signaling in inflammation and cancer. Molecular Cancer. 2013;**12**: 86

[82] Mitchell JP, Carmody RJ. NF-kappa B and the transcriptional control of inflammation. International Review of Cell and Molecular Biology. 2018;**335**: 41-84

[83] Abraham AC et al. Targeting the NF-kappa B signaling pathway in chronic tendon disease. Science Translational Medicine. 2019;**11**:eaav4319

[84] Loiselle AE et al. Development of antisense oligonucleotide (ASO) technology against Tgf-beta Signaling to prevent scarring during flexor tendon repair. Journal of Orthopaedic Research. 2015;**33**:859-866

[85] Zhang Y, Alexander PB, Wang XF. TGF-beta family Signaling in the control of cell proliferation and survival. Cold Spring Harbor Perspectives in Biology. 2017;**9**:a022145

[86] Jiang S et al. Down-regulating ERK1/2 and SMAD2/3 phosphorylation by physical barrier of celecoxib-loaded electrospun fibrous membranes prevents tendon adhesions. Biomaterials. 2014;**35**:9920-9929

[87] Yao Z et al. MicroRNA-21-3p engineered umbilical cord stem cell-derived exosomes inhibit tendon adhesion. Journal of Inflammation Research. 2020;**13**:303-316

[88] Yao Z et al. MicroRNA engineered umbilical cord stem cell-derived exosomes direct tendon regeneration by mTOR signaling. Journal of Nanobiotechnology. 2021;**19**:169

[89] Hata A, Chen YG. TGF-beta Signaling from receptors to Smads. Cold Spring Harbor Perspectives in Biology. 2016;**8**:a022061

[90] Wu G et al. Three-dimensional tendon scaffold loaded with TGF-beta1 gene silencing plasmid prevents tendon adhesion and promotes tendon repair. ACS Biomaterials Science & Engineering. 2021;**7**:5739-5748

[91] Weng CH et al. Interleukin-17A induces renal fibrosis through the ERK and Smad signaling pathways. Biomedicine & Pharmacotherapy. 2020;**123**:109741

[92] Wu B et al. The TGF-beta superfamily cytokine activin-a is induced during autoimmune neuroinflammation and drives pathogenic Th17 cell differentiation. Immunity. 2021;**54**:308-323 e306

[93] Katzel EB et al. Impact of Smad3 loss of function on scarring and adhesion formation during tendon healing. Journal of Orthopaedic Research. 2011;**29**:684-693

[94] Xue M et al. Endogenous MMP-9 and not MMP-2 promotes rheumatoid synovial fibroblast survival, inflammation and cartilage degradation. Rheumatology (Oxford, England). 2014;**53**:2270-2279

[95] Margulis A et al. MMP dependence of fibroblast contraction and collagen production induced by human mast cell activation in a three-dimensional collagen lattice. American Journal of Physiology. Lung Cellular and Molecular Physiology. 2009;**296**:L236-L247

[96] Loiselle AE et al. Remodeling of murine Intrasynovial tendon adhesions following injury: MMP and Neotendon gene expression. Journal of Orthopaedic Research. 2009;**27**:833-840

[97] Lu CC et al. Lateral slit delivery of bone marrow stromal cells enhances regeneration in the decellularized allograft flexor tendon. The Journal of Orthopaedic Translation. 2019;**19**:58-67

[98] Cai C et al. Self-healing hydrogel embodied with macrophage-regulation and responsive-gene-silencing properties for synergistic prevention of

peritendinous adhesion. Advanced Materials. 2022;**34**:e2106564

[99] Blomgran P, Blomgran R, Ernerudh J, Aspenberg P. Cox-2 inhibition and the composition of inflammatory cell populations during early and mid-time tendon healing. Muscle, Ligaments and Tendons Journal. 2017;**7**:223-229

[100] Cheng H et al. Role of prostaglandin E2 in tissue repair and regeneration. Theranostics. 2021;**11**: 8836-8854

[101] Dolkart O et al. Statins enhance rotator cuff healing by stimulating the COX2/PGE2/EP4 pathway an In vivo and In vitro study. The American Journal of Sports Medicine. 2014;**42**:2869-2876

[102] Wang Y et al. High concentration of aspirin induces apoptosis in rat tendon stem cells via inhibition of the Wnt/beta-catenin pathway. Cellular Physiology and Biochemistry. 2018;**50**:2046-2059

[103] Bindu S, Mazumder S, Bandyopadhyay U. Non-steroidal anti-inflammatory drugs (NSAIDs) and organ damage: A current perspective. Biochemical Pharmacology. 2020;**180**: 114147

[104] Guo C et al. Pharmacological properties and derivatives of shikonin-a review in recent years. Pharmacological Research. 2019;**149**:104463

[105] Geary MB et al. Systemic EP4 inhibition increases adhesion formation in a murine model of flexor tendon repair. PLoS One. 2015;**10**:e0136351

[106] Samora JB, Klinefelter RD. Flexor tendon reconstruction. The Journal of the American Academy of Orthopaedic Surgeons. 2016;**24**:28-36

[107] Malizos KN et al. Infections of deep hand and wrist compartments. Microorganisms. 2020;**8**:838

[108] Pickrell BB, Eberlin KR. Secondary surgery following replantation and revascularization. Hand Clinics. 2019;**35**: 231-240

[109] Shalumon KT et al. Multi-functional electrospun antibacterial core-shell nanofibrous membranes for prolonged prevention of post-surgical tendon adhesion and inflammation. Acta Biomaterialia. 2018;**72**:121-136

[110] Altan E, Yalcin L. Release of adhesions after zone II flexor tendon repair: The 'Gigli suture' technique. The Journal of Hand Surgery (European Volume). 2017;**42**:525-526

[111] Zhang CH et al. Evaluation of decellularized bovine tendon sheets for Achilles tendon defect reconstruction in a rabbit model. The American Journal of Sports Medicine. 2018;**46**:2687-2699

[112] Van der Merwe W et al. Xenograft for anterior cruciate ligament reconstruction was associated with high graft processing infection. The Journal of Experimental Orthopaedics. 2020;**7**:79

[113] Bai T, Zhang Q, Leng Y. A comparative study of biological and nonbiological sheath substitute in prevention of flexor tendon adhesions. Journal of Nanjing Railway Medical College. 1999;**18**:229-232

[114] Kulick MI, Brazlow R, Smith S, Hentz VR. Injectable ibuprofen: Preliminary evaluation of its ability to decrease peritendinous adhesions. Annals of Plastic Surgery. 1984;**13**: 459-467

[115] Moore N et al. Pharmacoepidemiology of non-steroidal

anti-inflammatory drugs. Thérapie. 2019;**74**:271-277

[116] McGrath MH. Local steroid therapy in the hand. The Journal of Hand Surgery. 1984;**9**:915-921

[117] Tatari H et al. Deleterious effects of local corticosteroid injections on the Achilles tendon of rats. Archives of Orthopaedic and Trauma Surgery. 2001; **121**:333-337

[118] Yu HL et al. RGD-peptides modifying dexamethasone: To enhance the anti-inflammatory efficacy and limit the risk of osteoporosis. MedChemComm. 2015;**6**:1345-1351

[119] Wu W et al. Advances in biomaterials for preventing tissue adhesion. Journal of Controlled Release. 2017;**261**:318-336

[120] Alimohammadi M et al. Electrospun nanofibrous membranes for preventing tendon adhesion. ACS Biomaterials Science & Engineering. 2020;**6**:4356-4376

[121] Khan F, Tanaka M. Designing smart biomaterials for tissue engineering. International Journal of Molecular Sciences. 2017;**19**:17

[122] Jenkins MJ, Harrison KL. The effect of crystalline morphology on the degradation of polycaprolactone in a solution of phosphate buffer and lipase. Polymers for Advanced Technologies. 2008;**19**:1901-1906

[123] Guo M et al. The effects of tensile stress on degradation of biodegradable PLGA membranes: A quantitative study. Polymer Degradation and Stability. 2016;**124**:95-100

[124] Migliaresi C, Fambri L, Cohn D. A study on the in vitro degradation of poly (lactic acid). Journal of Biomaterials Science. Polymer Edition. 1994;**5**: 591-606

[125] Goh JC, Sahoo S. Scaffolds for tendon and ligament tissue engineering. In: Regenerative Medicine and Biomaterials for the Repair of Connective Tissues. Sawston Cambridge, UK: Woodhead Publishing; 2010

[126] Cannella V et al. In vitro biocompatibility evaluation of nine dermal fillers on L929 cell line. BioMed Research International. 2020;**2020**: 8676343

[127] Chen SH, Chen CH, Fong YT, Chen JP. Prevention of peritendinous adhesions with electrospun chitosan-grafted polycaprolactone nanofibrous membranes. Acta Biomaterialia. 2014;**10**: 4971-4982

[128] Liu S et al. Prevention of peritendinous adhesions with electrospun ibuprofen-loaded poly(L-lactic acid)-polyethylene glycol fibrous membranes. Tissue Engineering. Part A. 2013;**19**:529-537

[129] Uyanik O et al. Prevention of peritendinous adhesions with electrospun poly (lactic acid-co-glycolic acid) (PLGA) bioabsorbable nanofiber: An experimental study. Colloids and Surfaces. B, Biointerfaces. 2022;**209**: 112181

[130] Song A, Rane AA, Christman KL. Antibacterial and cell-adhesive polypeptide and poly(ethylene glycol) hydrogel as a potential scaffold for wound healing. Acta Biomaterialia. 2012; **8**:41-50

[131] Karaaltin MV et al. The effects of 5-fluorouracil on flexor tendon healing by using a biodegradable gelatin, slow

releasing system: Experimental study in a hen model. The Journal of Hand Surgery (European Volume). 2013;**38**: 651-657

[132] Moreland LW. Intra-articular hyaluronan (hyaluronic acid) and hylans for the treatment of osteoarthritis: Mechanisms of action. Arthritis Research & Therapy. 2003;**5**:54-67

[133] Yilmaz E et al. The effect of seprafilm on adhesion formation and tendon healing after flexor tendon repair in chicken. Orthopedics. 2010;**33**: 164-170

[134] Kuo SM et al. Evaluation of the ability of xanthan gum/gellan gum/ hyaluronan hydrogel membranes to prevent the adhesion of postrepaired tendons. Carbohydrate Polymers. 2014; **114**:230-237

[135] Burgisser GM, Buschmann J. History and performance of implant materials applied as peritendinous antiadhesives. Journal of Biomedical Materials Research Part B. 2015;**103**: 212-228

[136] Ishiyama N et al. Reduction of peritendinous adhesions by hydrogel containing biocompatible phospholipid polymer MPC for tendon repair. The Journal of Bone and Joint Surgery. American Volume. 2011;**93**: 142-149

[137] Liu R, Zhang S, Chen X. Injectable hydrogels for tendon and ligament tissue engineering. Journal of Tissue Engineering and Regenerative Medicine. 2020;**14**:1333-1348

[138] Chou PY et al. Thermo-responsive in-situ forming hydrogels as barriers to prevent post-operative peritendinous adhesion. Acta Biomaterialia. 2017;**63**: 85-95

[139] Zhou YL et al. Localized delivery of miRNAs targets cyclooxygenases and reduces flexor tendon adhesions. Acta Biomaterialia. 2018;**70**:237-248

[140] Rinoldi C et al. Mechanical and biochemical stimulation of 3D multilayered scaffolds for tendon tissue engineering. ACS Biomaterials Science & Engineering. 2019;**5**:2953-2964

[141] Madkhali O, Mekhail G, Wettig SD. Modified gelatin nanoparticles for gene delivery. International Journal of Pharmaceutics. 2019;**554**:224-234

[142] Lee EJ, Kasper FK, Mikos AG. Biomaterials for tissue engineering. Annals of Biomedical Engineering. 2014; **42**:323-337

[143] Lomas AJ et al. The past, present and future in scaffold-based tendon treatments. Advanced Drug Delivery Reviews. 2015;**84**:257-277

[144] James R, Kesturu G, Balian G, Chhabra AB. Tendon: Biology, biomechanics, repair, growth factors, and evolving treatment options. The Journal of Hand Surgery. 2008;**33**: 102-112

[145] Zhou YL, Yang QQ, Zhang L, Tang JB. Nanoparticle-coated sutures providing sustained growth factor delivery to improve the healing strength of injured tendons. Acta Biomaterialia. 2021;**124**:301-314

[146] Liu S et al. Biomimetic sheath membrane via electrospinning for antiadhesion of repaired tendon. Biomacromolecules. 2012;**13**:3611-3619

[147] Yao Y et al. Effect of sustained heparin release from PCL/chitosan hybrid small-diameter vascular grafts on anti-thrombogenic property and

endothelialization. Acta Biomaterialia. 2014;**10**:2739-2749

[148] Zhang Q et al. Electrospun polymeric micro/nanofibrous scaffolds for long-term drug release and their biomedical applications. Drug Discovery Today. 2017;**22**:1351-1366

[149] Luong-Van E et al. Controlled release of heparin from poly(epsilon-caprolactone) electrospun fibers. Biomaterials. 2006;**27**:2042-2050

[150] Szentivanyi A, Chakradeo T, Zernetsch H, Glasmacher B. Electrospun cellular microenvironments: Understanding controlled release and scaffold structure. Advanced Drug Delivery Reviews. 2011;**63**:209-220

[151] Casper CL, Yamaguchi N, Kiick KL, Rabolt JF. Functionalizing electrospun fibers with biologically relevant macromolecules. Biomacromolecules. 2005;**6**:1998-2007

[152] Zeng J et al. Poly(vinyl alcohol) nanofibers by electrospinning as a protein delivery system and the retardation of enzyme release by additional polymer coatings. Biomacromolecules. 2005;**6**: 1484-1488

[153] Zomer Volpato F et al. Preservation of FGF-2 bioactivity using heparin-based nanoparticles, and their delivery from electrospun chitosan fibers. Acta Biomaterialia. 2012;**8**:1551-1559

[154] Cheng L et al. Surface biofunctional drug-loaded electrospun fibrous scaffolds for comprehensive repairing hypertrophic scars. Biomaterials. 2016; **83**:169-181

[155] Sultanova Z, Kaleli G, Kabay G, Mutlu M. Controlled release of a hydrophilic drug from coaxially electrospun polycaprolactone nanofibers. International Journal of Pharmaceutics. 2016;**505**:133-138

[156] Jiang YN, Mo HY, Yu DG. Electrospun drug-loaded core-sheath PVP/zein nanofibers for biphasic drug release. International Journal of Pharmaceutics. 2012;**438**:232-239

[157] Hu J et al. Drug-loaded emulsion electrospun nanofibers: Characterization, drug release and in vitro biocompatibility. RSC Advances. 2015;**5**:100256-100267

[158] Sy JC, Klemm AS, Shastri VP. Emulsion as a means of controlling electrospinning of polymers. Advanced Materials. 2009;**21**:376-381

[159] Zhao X et al. Optimization of intrinsic and extrinsic tendon healing through controllable water-soluble mitomycin-C release from electrospun fibers by mediating adhesion-related gene expression. Biomaterials. 2015;**61**: 61-74

[160] Xu X et al. Ultrafine medicated fibers electrospun from W/O emulsions. Journal of Controlled Release. 2005;**108**: 33-42

[161] Manning CN et al. Controlled delivery of mesenchymal stem cells and growth factors using a nanofiber scaffold for tendon repair. Acta Biomaterialia. 2013;**9**:6905-6914

[162] Chainani A et al. Multilayered electrospun scaffolds for tendon tissue engineering. Tissue Engineering. Part A. 2013;**19**:2594-2604

[163] Li LF et al. Release of celecoxib from a bi-layer biomimetic tendon sheath to prevent tissue adhesion. Materials Science and Engineering C:

Materials for Biological Applications. 2016;**61**:220-226

[164] Okuda T, Tominaga K, Kidoaki S. Time-programmed dual release formulation by multilayered drug-loaded nanofiber meshes. Journal of Controlled Release. 2010;**143**:258-264

[165] Hu C, Cui W. Hierarchical structure of electrospun composite fibers for long-term controlled drug release carriers. Advanced Healthcare Materials. 2012;**1**:809-814

[166] Hu C et al. Long-term drug release from electrospun fibers for in vivo inflammation prevention in the prevention of peritendinous adhesions. Acta Biomaterialia. 2013;**9**:7381-7388

[167] Slowing II, Vivero-Escoto JL, Wu CW, Lin VS. Mesoporous silica nanoparticles as controlled release drug delivery and gene transfection carriers. Advanced Drug Delivery Reviews. 2008;**60**:1278-1288

[168] Kim CH et al. An improved hydrophilicity via electrospinning for enhanced cell attachment and proliferation. Journal of Biomedical Materials Research. Part B, Applied Biomaterials. 2006;**78**:283-290

[169] De Bartolo L, Morelli S, Bader A, Drioli E. The influence of polymeric membrane surface free energy on cell metabolic functions. Journal of Materials Science. Materials in Medicine. 2001;**12**:959-963

[170] Fakhraei O et al. Nanofibrous polycaprolactone/chitosan membranes for preventing postsurgical tendon adhesion. Journal of Biomedical Materials Research. Part B, Applied Biomaterials. 2022;**110**:1279-1291

[171] Van der Schueren L, Steyaert I, De Schoenmaker B, De Clerck K. Polycaprolactone/chitosan blend nanofibres electrospun from an acetic acid/formic acid solvent system. Carbohydrate Polymers. 2012;**88**:1221-1226

[172] Wang YW et al. Effect of mitomycin on normal dermal fibroblast and HaCat cell: An in vitro study. Journal of Zhejiang University. Science. B. 2012;**13**:997-1005

[173] Chen CH, Chen SH, Shalumon KT, Chen JP. Dual functional core-sheath electrospun hyaluronic acid/polycaprolactone nanofibrous membranes embedded with silver nanoparticles for prevention of peritendinous adhesion. Acta Biomaterialia. 2015;**26**:225-235

[174] Chen CH et al. Functional hyaluronic acid-polylactic acid/silver nanoparticles Core-sheath nanofiber membranes for prevention of post-operative tendon adhesion. International Journal of Molecular Sciences. 2021;**22**:8781

[175] El Khatib M et al. Fabrication and plasma surface activation of aligned electrospun PLGA Fiber fleeces with improved adhesion and infiltration of amniotic epithelial stem cells maintaining their Teno-inductive potential. Molecules. 2020;**25**:3176

[176] Liu S et al. Tendon healing and anti-adhesion properties of electrospun fibrous membranes containing bFGF loaded nanoparticles. Biomaterials. 2013;**34**:4690-4701

[177] Liao JCY et al. The effects of bi-functional anti-adhesion scaffolds on flexor tendon healing in a rabbit model. Journal of Biomedical Materials

Research. Part B, Applied Biomaterials. 2018;**106**:2605-2614

[178] Liu S et al. Gene silencing via PDA/ERK2-siRNA-mediated electrospun Fibers for peritendinous antiadhesion. Advanced Science (Weinheim, Baden-Württemberg, Germany). 2019;**6**: 1801217

[179] Li F et al. Efficient inhibition of the formation of joint adhesions by ERK2 small interfering RNAs. Biochemical and Biophysical Research Communications. 2010;**391**:795-799

[180] Tang JB et al. Gene therapy strategies to improve strength and quality of flexor tendon healing. Expert Opinion on Biological Therapy. 2016;**16**: 291-301

[181] Liu S et al. Macrophage infiltration of electrospun polyester fibers. Biomaterials Science. 2017;**5**:1579-1587

[182] Chen E et al. An asymmetric chitosan scaffold for tendon tissue engineering. Acta Biomaterialia. 2018;**73**: 377-387

[183] Jayasree A et al. Bioengineered braided micro-nano (multiscale) fibrous scaffolds for tendon reconstruction. ACS Biomaterials Science & Engineering. 2019;**11**:1476-1486

[184] Park DY et al. Cross-linked cartilage acellular matrix film decreases postsurgical peritendinous adhesions. Artificial Organs. 2020;**44**:E136-E149

[185] Song Y et al. Surface modification of electrospun fibers with mechano-growth factor for mitigating the foreign-body reaction. Bioactive Materials. 2021;**6**: 2983-2998

[186] Liu YS et al. No midterm advantages in the middle term using small intestinal submucosa and human amniotic membrane in Achilles tendon transverse tenotomy. Journal of Orthopaedic Surgery and Research. 2016;**11**:125

[187] Koob TJ et al. Biological properties of dehydrated human amnion/chorion composite graft: Implications for chronic wound healing. International Wound Journal. 2013;**10**:493-500

[188] Dogramaci Y, Duman IG. Reinforcement of the flexor tendon repair using human amniotic MembraneA biomechanical evaluation using the modified Kessler method of tendon repair. Journal of the American Podiatric Medical Association. 2016;**106**: 319-322

[189] Liu C et al. Experimental study of tendon sheath repair via decellularized amnion to prevent tendon adhesion. PLoS One. 2018;**13**:e0205811

[190] Prakash S, Kalra P, Dhal A. Flexor tendon repair with amniotic membrane. International Orthopaedics. 2020;**44**: 2037-2045

[191] Bennett NT, Schultz GS. Growth-factors and wound-healing—Biochemical-properties of growth-factors and their receptors. American Journal of Surgery. 1993;**165**:728-737

[192] Shu J et al. Human amnion mesenchymal cells inhibit lipopolysaccharide-induced TNF-alpha and IL-1beta production in THP-1 cells. Biological Research. 2015;**48**:69

[193] Duan-Arnold Y et al. Retention of endogenous viable cells enhances the anti-inflammatory activity of cryopreserved amnion. Advances in Wound Care (New Rochelle). 2015;**4**: 523-533

[194] Yao M et al. Phototoxicity is not associated with photochemical tissue bonding of skin. Lasers in Surgery and Medicine. 2010;**42**:123-131

[195] Liu CJ et al. Regulation of ERK1/2 and SMAD2/3 pathways by using multi-layered electrospun PCL-amnion nanofibrous membranes for the prevention of post-surgical tendon adhesion. International Journal of Nanomedicine. 2020;**15**:927-942

[196] Liu C et al. Biological amnion prevents flexor tendon adhesion in zone II: A controlled, multicentre clinical trial. BioMed Research International. **2019**; **2019**:2354325

[197] Leppanen OV et al. Outcomes after flexor tendon repair combined with the application of human amniotic membrane allograft. The Journal of Hand Surgery. 2017;**42**:474 e471-474 e478

[198] Kibadi K, Moutet F. Silicone infusion tubing instead of hunter rods for two-stage zone 2 flexor tendon reconstruction in a resource-limited surgical environment. Hand Surgery & Rehabilitation. 2017;**36**:384-387

[199] Sedghizadeh P et al. Design and in vivo testing of novel bisphosphonate-fluoroquinolone conjugates chemisorbed to bone graft material. Journal of Bone and Mineral Research. 2019;**34**:367-368

[200] Moshiri A, Oryan A, Meimandi-Parizi A. Synthesis, development, characterization and effectiveness of bovine pure platelet gel-collagen-polydioxanone bioactive graft on tendon healing. Journal of Cellular and Molecular Medicine. 2015;**19**:1308-1332

[201] Harvey T, Flamenco S, Fan CM. A Tppp3(+)Pdgfra(+) tendon stem cell population contributes to regeneration and reveals a shared role for PDGF signalling in regeneration and fibrosis. Nature Cell Biology. 2019;**21**:1490-1503

[202] Al-Qattan MM. Two-staged extensor tendon reconstruction for zone 6 extensor tendon loss of the fingers: Indications, technique and results. The Journal of Hand Surgery (European Volume). 2015;**40**:276-280

[203] Sundine M, Scheker LR. A comparison of immediate and staged reconstruction of the dorsum of the hand. Journal of Hand Surgery (British). 1996;**21**:216-221

[204] Adani R, Marcoccio I, Tarallo L. Flap coverage of dorsum of hand associated with extensor tendons injuries: A completely vascularized single-stage reconstruction. Microsurgery. 2003;**23**:32-39

[205] Abdulaziz MKB et al. Two-stage reconstruction of hand extensor tendons using silicon rods. Plastic and Reconstructive Surgery—Global Open. 2021;**9**:e3858

[206] Bashaireh KM, Audat Z, Radaideh AM, Aleshawi AJ. The effectiveness of autograft used in anterior cruciate ligament reconstruction of the knee: Surgical Records for the new Generations of Orthopedic surgeons and synthetic graft revisit. Orthopedic Research and Reviews. 2020;**12**:61-67

[207] Satora W, Krolikowska A, Czamara A, Reichert P. Synthetic grafts in the treatment of ruptured anterior cruciate ligament of the knee joint. Polimery w Medycynie. 2017;**47**:55-59

[208] Seiler JG 3rd et al. The Marshall R. Urist Young Investigator Award. Autogenous flexor tendon grafts. Biologic mechanisms for incorporation.

Clinical Orthopaedics and Related Research. 1997;**345**:239-247

[209] Berglund M et al. Assessment of mRNA levels for matrix molecules and TGF- beta1 in rabbit flexor and peroneus tendons reveals regional differences in steady-state expression. Journal of Hand Surgery (British). 2004;**29**:165-169

[210] Peacock EE Jr, Madden JW. Human composite flexor tendon allografts. Annals of Surgery. 1967;**166**:624-629

[211] Drake DB, Tilt AC, DeGeorge BR. Acellular flexor tendon allografts: A new horizon for tendon reconstruction. The Journal of Hand Surgery. 2013;**38**:2491-2495

[212] DeGeorge BR Jr, Rodeheaver GT, Drake DB. The biophysical characteristics of human composite flexor tendon allograft for upper extremity reconstruction. Annals of Plastic Surgery. 2014;**72**:S184-S190

[213] Kryger GS et al. A comparison of tenocytes and mesenchymal stem cells for use in flexor tendon tissue engineering. The Journal of Hand Surgery. 2007;**32a**:597-605

[214] Basile P et al. Freeze-dried tendon Allografts as tissue-engineering scaffolds for gdf5 gene delivery. Molecular Therapy. 2008;**16**:466-473

[215] Zhao C et al. Improvement of flexor tendon reconstruction with carbodiimide-derivatized hyaluronic acid and gelatin-modified intrasynovial allografts: Study of a primary repair failure model. The Journal of Bone and Joint Surgery. American Volume. 2010; **92**:2817-2828

[216] Tang L et al. Long-term effectiveness of tendon allograft for repairing tendon defect. Zhongguo Xiu Fu Chong Jian Wai Ke Za Zhi. 2011;**25**: 341-343

[217] Baymurat AC et al. Bio-engineered synovial membrane to prevent tendon adhesions in rabbit flexor tendon model. Journal of Biomedical Materials Research. Part A. 2015;**103**:84-90

[218] Sungur N et al. Prevention of tendon adhesions by the reconstruction of the tendon sheath with solvent dehydrated bovine pericard: An experimental study. The Journal of Trauma. 2006;**61**:1467-1472

Section 4

Insights for Treatment

Chapter 4

Medical Implications of the Relationships among Protein Denaturation, Necrosis and Inflammation: An Intriguing Story

Bruno Silvestrini and Mauro Silvestrini

Abstract

This story deals with the role of protein denaturation in inflammation. The starting point was the description of the necrotizing action of inflammatory proteins, followed by the discovery of the antidenaturant action of NSAIDs (nonsteroidal anti-inflammatory drugs). Hence, the idea is that the antidenaturant action accounted for the action of NSAIDs. This hypothesis was dropped following the discovery of the antiprostaglandin action of NSAIDs, which shifted the focus to the arachidonic acid cascade. It was revived by assuming that protein denaturation is a process in its own, suitable for separate medical treatment. This approach led to bendazac and bindarit, the first selective antidenaturant drugs. This experience shows that protein denaturation has two main pathological sequelae. The first concerns the so-called primary (innate) inflammation. The second sequela concerns the so-called secondary (acquired) inflammation. Natural antidenaturant agents represent a promising alternative to the synthetics bendazac and bindarit. Within this framework, tendinitis finds a separate but significant place.

Keywords: inflammation, protein denaturation, bendazac, bindarit, fatty acids, tendons

1. Introduction

To start with, inflammation is part of homeostasis, the fundamental process of life of preserving the milieu intérieur by reacting to changes with opposing measures [1–3]. More specifically, inflammation is "the vital response to injury", which may be related to exposure to infection, toxins, damaged cells, waste, and chemical and physical agents [4, 5]. The function of inflammation is to repair the damage that does not result from the inflammation itself, but from overactivation or deviation of the underlying physiological process. Consider the five cardinal signs of inflammation described by Celsius and Galen over 2000 years ago: heat (calor), pain (dolor), redness (rubor), swelling (tumor), and impairment (functio laesa). Without pain, for example, a person would be exposed to disease without realizing it. Similarly, impairment (functio laesa) implies the setting aside of a function to allow recovery. A fracture would not be repaired without temporary immobilization of the broken bone. The overlap of physiological and pathological elements is the key point of the medical treatment of inflammation. Based on these introductory remarks, there are two inflammatory processes. The innate one is based on the hyperactivation of genetically innate physiological processes. Acquired inflammation is different in that it involves the immune system.

2. Pathophysiological considerations

It consists of an immune reaction adapted to each aggressive agent so as to neutralize it without damaging the surrounding tissues. This measure takes into account the genetic characteristics that distinguish each living being, as well as the chemical structure and macromolecules that the organism must take up. Acquired inflammation combines the collateral damage of innate and acquired processes. For example, deaths from SARS-CoV-2 and variants are caused not only by the virus, which penetrates and kills cells but also by the excessive immune-inflammatory reaction that impairs respiration and blood clotting.

With this in mind, the current story begins about 60 years ago with the description of the irritating and necrotizing effects on the skin of protein complexes related to both acquired and innate inflammation [6–9]. It should be noted that a similar necrotizing effect is produced by urea, a metabolite of the aforementioned complexes [10]. Subsequently, NSAIDs were found to exert an antidenaturant action at concentrations that roughly correspond to their anti-inflammatory effects [11, 12]. The resulting hypothesis was that "most strongly anti-inflammatory drugs might owe at least part of their effects on some biochemical processes to their physicochemical property of interacting with proteins." The quoted portion is from the original article [12]. Simply put, the hypothesis was that the antidenaturant effect of NSAIDs underlies their mechanism of action. Hence, the protein denaturation assay was proposed as a simple screening test for antirheumatic and antiphlogistic drugs [13, 14]. The protein-centered hypothesis had some inconsistencies. For example, the antidenaturant effect occurs at relatively higher concentrations than at anti-inflammatory concentrations [15]. In addition, antidenaturant drugs may not have anti-inflammatory effects [16].

Inconsistencies aside, the above hypothesis was abandoned following the discovery of the antiprostaglandin action of aspirin-like drugs, which shifted the focus to the arachidonic acid cascade [17]. Prostaglandins are lipid autacoids derived from arachidonic acid that have widespread physiological roles in the body, including homeostatic functions involved in the inflammatory process [18]. The arachidonic acid cascade fits like a glove with the concept that inflammation involves the hyperactivation of a physiological process. For example, NSAIDs reduce mucosal hypersecretion in the common cold, along with a reduction in the physiological secretion that protects the gastric mucosa [19]. In fact, it has been reported that half of the patients treated with NSAIDs have gastric erosions and 10–30% have gastric ulcers [20]. Therefore, the problem of overlap between physiological and pathological aspects of inflammation has remained unresolved.

Incidentally, steroidal anti-inflammatory drugs are different. Rather than showing antidenaturant and antiprostaglandin effects, they inhibit the functions of leukocytes, which participate in both innate and acquired inflammation [21]. Their mechanism of action is reminiscent of the stress "attack" reaction to dangerous and life-threatening events [22, 23]. This reaction consists of a threefold adrenal discharge involving sympathetic catecholamines, glucocorticosteroids, and mineralcorticostseroids [24, 25]. Leukocyte functions [including the immune response] are temporarily set aside, as they are useless in acute emergencies. In essence, adrenal discharge activates the somatic and mental processes needed to cope with emergencies. During World War II, the Nazis administered an adrenal cortex extract to fighter pilots that mimicked the corresponding biological process. Steroidal anti-inflammatory drugs belong to the above stress discharge, including hydrocortisone (cortisol), which has been found to explain the remission of jaundice-induced rheumatoid arthritis [26, 27]. We will return to this phenomenon shortly.

Returning to the protein-centered inflammation hypothesis, it has been revived in different terms. The idea was that protein denaturation was a process in its own right, suitable for separate medical treatment [28, 29]. Similarly, paracetamol is an anti-inflammatory drug that shows selective antinociceptive and antifebrile effects. Based on this idea, the aforementioned protein denaturation assay [13, 14] was used to select drugs, with the exception that they had to be free of the antiphlogistic and related side effects that others sought.

3. Pharmacotherapeutic implications

Bendazac, also known as bendazolic acid, is the first selective antidenaturant drug that has undergone thorough preclinical evaluation and medical use. The drug teaches something about the theoretical and practical value of this approach. First, the antidenaturant action of bendazac is against several agents, including extreme pH, heat, UV, and sunlight [10, 30–34]. It follows that bendazac is not a free radical scavenger. Rather, it binds to reactive protein sites, thus providing a protective barrier against free radicals. This binding does not result in a significant change in protein architecture and function. This suggests that the antidenaturant action depends on Van der Waals forces, which differ from covalent and ionic forces. Rather, they depend on the fluctuating polarizations of neighboring particles as a consequence of quantum dynamics.

Considering the pharmacological profile of bendazac, its most striking feature is its antinecrotic action [10]. Therefore, clinical studies have focused on dystrophic conditions [35]. More specifically, bendazac has been tested and shown to be active against inflammatory and allergic dermatoses: contact dermatitis, occupational dermatitis, seborrheic dermatitis, diaper and childhood dermatitis, constitutional eczema, erythema and localized itching, urticaria, drug allergies, and insect bites [36–42].

Thus, the preclinical and clinical experience gathered with bendazac supported the idea that protein denaturation is a process in its own right, suitable for targeted medical treatment. It is noteworthy that bendazac has been shown to be active against cataracts, which consist of physical opacification of the lens [43–46]. This suggests that a protein-denaturing agent could affect other medical conditions, such as kidney and gallstones, which are triggered by a protein-denaturing core.

Bindarit is another selective antidenaturant drug [47]. It shares a pharmacological profile with bendazac, but its study focused on adjuvant-induced arthritis in rats. It consists of the injection of Freund's adjuvant (a fine suspension of dead tubercle bacilli in liquid kerosene) into the plantar pad of rats. The adjuvant produces a primary inflammatory lesion at the injection site, followed, after about 10–15 days, by secondary lesions in areas of the body distant from the injection site [48–51]. The secondary lesions are accompanied by humoral changes consisting of denatured

GLIMBAL-like (globulin-like migrating proteins) proteins, which have been detected in patients with rheumatoid arthritis [52]. Returning to bindarit, it selectively inhibits secondary lesions and related humoral changes, whereas hydrocortisone- and aspirin-like drugs inhibit both primary and secondary lesions [47]. Subsequently, bindarit was found to prolong survival and reduce renal damage in murine autoimmune disease [53, 54]. At this point, available information suggests that: (A) protein denaturation triggers the secondary immune-inflammatory process by exposing antigens common to both denatured and native proteins; and (B) an antidenaturing drug may show a protective action against autoimmune conditions in the absence of immunosuppressive effects. The resulting medical opportunities are exciting, but nevertheless, after 20 years bindarit still remains a matter of preclinical research and working hypotheses. Why?

The answer deserves a separate comment. It goes back to 1961, the year of thalidomide when images of phocomelic infants went around the world. This tragedy sent a warning signal about the risks of the hitherto uncontrolled use of synthetic drugs. Since then, they have been subject to strict toxicological controls, which have increased safety but burdened and delayed medical use. At the same time, there has been a resurgence of interest in drugs of natural origin, such as hormones, vitamins, and vaccines. They are not necessarily safer than synthetic ones, but they have a history of how to use them safely.

"It is important for us to identify nature's powerful, if accidental, antidotes," said Philip Hench on the occasion of receiving the Nobel Prize for the discovery of hydrocortisone. A small but exciting opportunity in the field of natural antidotes came with the experimental reevaluation of jaundice, the natural phenomenon that had paved the way for the treatment of rheumatoid arthritis with hydrocortisone a quarter century earlier [26, 27]. In a nutshell, it was discovered that jaundice involves an inhibition of protein denaturation, which, based on the above data and ideas, could participate in the remission of rheumatoid arthritis [55]. This phenomenon was partly attributable to the antidenaturant bilirubin and bile salts, but the effective doses and concentrations were hardly compatible with medical use. Hence, the search for more convenient compounds. Among the natural substances examined so far [56–60], candidates for medical use include fatty acids belonging to the composition of cell membranes [61]. Like bile salts and bendazac, they also prevent hemolysis of erythrocytes [62–64]. Hopefully, they will not have the same fate as bindarit.

In this story focusing on protein denaturation, tendinitis occupies a marginal but significant position. The tendon consists mainly of collagen (80%), the most abundant, ubiquitous, and versatile protein in mammals [65]. The type I collagen in the tendon gives it the strength and elasticity needed to connect muscle to bone, transmitting the mechanical forces of muscle contraction to the skeletal system. Its denaturation results in a loss of its elastoplastic function, which is irreversible. Experience with collagen deficiency disease suggests that tendinitis could also be addressed with dietary measures that promote collagen regeneration [66]. This is the message of the biological evidence, which is different but sometimes as strong as the experimental evidence.

4. Conclusions

This long and intriguing story ends up under the banner of biology. In modern science, it has been pushed aside by molecular biology, which focuses on single details that are difficult to trace back to their overall meaning. It is a kind of intellectual,

DOI: http://dx.doi.org/10.5772/intechopen.108018

rather than visual, myopia. Like the cells in which they are produced, proteins have a biological cycle: they are born, mature, age (denature) and disintegrate, giving rise to waste. Slags are normally recycled to synthesize new proteins that replace aged ones or are excreted. The problem of slag mainly affects so-called perennial cells, including lens cells and neurons that last a long time without renewing themselves and their proteins [67, 68]. This is the case with cataracts, which are caused by scoriae that blur vision. Bendazac shows that an antidenaturing agent could influence this condition by reducing the extent of protein denaturation [30]. Slag is also involved in brain proteinopathy, which is related to beta-amyloid denaturation resulting in the formation of aggregates and toxic metabolites [69, 70]. The use of high doses of aspirin, an antidenaturant, has been reported to reduce the prevalence of Alzheimer's dementia [71]. Unfortunately, NSAIDs are burdened with unavoidable side effects. Bendazac and bindarit are potentially a step forward because of their selective antidenaturant action. This article presents some additional natural compounds, which belong to the composition and apparently to the physiological modulation of the protein life cycle.

Author details

Bruno Silvestrini[1]* and Mauro Silvestrini[2]

1 The Noopolis Foundation, Rome, Italy

2 Department of Experimental and Clinical Medicine, Polytechnic University of Marche, Ancona, Italy

*Address all correspondence to: brunosilvestrini25@gmail.com

References

[1] Guyton AC. Medical Physiology. Philadelphia: Saunders; 1986

[2] Bernard C. Lectures on the Phenomena of Life Common to Animals and Plants. Springfield, Ill: Charles C Thomas Pub Ltd; 1974

[3] Cannon WB. Share on the body physiologic and the body politicy. Science. 1941;**93**(2401):1-10. DOI: 10.1126/science.93.240

[4] Robbins, Cotran. Pathologic Basis of Disease. 9th ed. Philadelphia, Saunders; 2015

[5] Lawyer's Guide to Forensic Medicine. Bernard Knight. Taylor & Francis Ed.; 2003

[6] Ishizaka K, Campbell DH. Biological activity of soluble antigen-antibody complexes. I. Skin reactive properties. Proceedings of the Society for Experimental Biology and Medicine. 1958;**97**(3):635-638. DOI: 10.3181/00379727-97-23829

[7] Ishizaka K, Ishizaka T, Campbell DH. The biological activity of soluble antigen-antibody complexes. II. Physical properties of soluble complexes having skin-irritating activity. Journal of Experimental Medicine. 1959;**109**(2): 127-143. DOI: 10.1084/jem.109.2.127

[8] Opie EL. On the relation of necrosis and inflammation to denaturation of proteins. The Journal of Experimental Medicine. 1962;**115**(3):597-608. DOI: 10.1084/jem.115.3.597

[9] Opie EL. The relation of inflammation to the molecular structure of carbon compounds soluble in the fluids of the body. The Journal of Experimental Medicine. 1965;**121**(4):487-501. DOI: 10.1084/jem.121.4.487

[10] Silvestrini B, Cioli V, Burberi S. Pharmacological properties of bendazac (AF 983) with particular reference to its topical action on some experimental inflammatory processes. Arzneimittel-Forschung. 1969;**19**(1):30-36

[11] Mizushima Y. Inhibition of protein denaturation by antirheumatic or antiphlogistic agents. Archives Internationales de Pharmacodynamie et de Therapie. 1964;**149**:1.0

[12] Mizushima Y. Effect of nonsteroidal anti-inflammatory drugs on proteins. In: Silvestrini B, Tura S, Spector WG, editors. Inflammation. Aetiopatogenetic, Clinical and Therapeutic Problems. Excerpta Medica Foundation; 1968

[13] Mizushima Y. Simple screening test for antirheumatic drugs. Lancet. 1965;**1**:169

[14] Mizushima Y. Screening test for antirheumatic drugs. Lancet. 1966;**288**:443

[15] Whitehouse MW. Some biochemical and pharmacological properties of antinflammatory drugs. Progress in Drug Research. 1965;**8**:321

[16] Del Basso OP, e Silvestrini B. Effetti di alcune sostanze sulla risposta turbidimetrica al calore dell'albumina e del siero e plasma di ratto. Giornale di Biochimica. 1966;**15**(3):198-212

[17] Vane J. Inhibition of prostaglandin synthesis as a mechanism of action for aspirin-like drugs. Nature New Biology. 1971;**231**:232-235. DOI: 10.1038/newbio231232a0

[18] Ricciotti E, FitzGerald GA. Prostaglandins and inflammation.

Arteriosclerosis, Thrombosis, and Vascular Biology. 2011;**31**(5):986-1000. DOI: 10.1161/ATVBAHA.110.207449

[19] Hawkey CJ. Non-steroidal anti-inflammatory drug gastropathy: causes and treatment. Scandinavian Journal of Gastroenterology. Supplement. 1996;**220**:124-127. DOI: 10.3109/00365529609094763

[20] Laine L. Nonsteroidal anti-inflammatory drug gastropathy. Gastrointestinal Endoscopy Clinics of North America. 1996;**6**(3):489-504

[21] Chrousos GP. The hypothalamic-pituitary-adrenal axis and immune-mediated inflammation. The New England Journal of Medicine. 1995;**332**(20):1351-1362. DOI: 10.1056/NEJM199505183322008

[22] Cannon WB. Bodily Changes in Pain, Hunger, Fear, and Rage. New York: Appleton-Century-Crofts; 1915. p. 211

[23] Silvestrini B. Drug Sickness. LAMBERT Academic Publishing; 2014. p. 52. See also Malati di droga. Lyra libri, Como (2011). P.57

[24] Segerstrom SC, Miller GE. Psychological stress and the human immune system: A meta-analytic study of 30 years of inquiry. Psychological Bulletin. 2004;**130**(4):601-630. DOI: 10.1037/0033-2909.130.4.601

[25] Padgett DA, Glaser R. How stress influences the immune response. Trends in Immunology. 2003;**24**(8):444-448. DOI: 10.1016/s1471-4906(03)00173-x

[26] Hench PS. Effect of spontaneous jaundice on rheumatoid (atrophic) arthritis attempts to reproduce the phenomenon. The British Medical Journal. 1938;**2**(4050):394-398 Available from: http://www.jstor.org/stable/20300483

[27] Hench PS, Kendall EC, et al. The effect of a hormone of the adrenal cortex (17-hydroxy-11-dehydrocorticosterone, compound E) and of pituitary adrenocorticotropic hormone on rheumatoid arthritis. Proceedings of the Staff Meetings. Mayo Clinic. 1949;**24**(8):181-197

[28] Silvestrini B. Primary and secondary inflammation. Panminerva Medica. 1969;**11**:587-593

[29] Silvestrini B. Working hypothesis exploited in the pharmacologic research of some anti-inflammatory agents. In: Silvestrini B, Tura S, Spector WG, editors. Inflammation. Aetiopatogenetic, Clinical and Therapeutic Problems. Excerpta Medica Foundation; 1968

[30] Silvestrini B, Catanese B, Lisciani R. A biochemical basis of the anti-inflammatory activity of Bendazac (AF 983). In: Bertelli A, Houck JC, editors. Inflammation Biochemistry and Drug Interaction. Amsterdam: Excerpta Med. Foundation; 1969. pp. 283-288

[31] Silvestrini B, Catanese B, Lisciani R, Alessandroni A. Studies on the mechanism of action of bendazac (AF 983). Arzneimittel Forschung. 1970;**20**:250-253

[32] Lisciani R, Scorza Barcellona P, Silvestrini B. Topical activity of Bendazac on experimental burns. Japan Journal of Pharmacology. 1971;**21**:69-73

[33] Silvestrini B, Catanese B, Lisciani R. Pharmacology of Bendazac. In: New Trends in Skin Therapeutics. Non-Steroid Anti-Inflammatory Local Treatment. Eds.: Fuga GC, De Gregorio M, Milbradt R. Roma: Leonardo Ediz. Sci.; 1975. pp. 1-9

[34] Scorza Barcellona P, Campana A, Caranti S, D'Onofrio E, Silvestrini B. Pre-treatment with bendazac attenuates retinal damage induced by intense light in rats. Pharmaceutical Research. 1991;**24**(1):105-112

[35] Zar E, De Gregorio M. Clinical evaluation of a new topical anti-inflammatory agent: Bendazolic acid (bendazac). Archivio di Chirurgia Toracica e Cardiovascolare. 1962;**5**(4):217-218

[36] Giacometti C, Dani F. Bendazolic acid in the therapy of some dermatoses. Clinical studies. G Italic Dermatology Minerva Dermatology. 1971;**46**(5):236-241

[37] Fuga GC, Proto A. Clinical considerations on a controlled trial of bendazolic acid in some dermatoses. G Italic Dermatology Minerva Dermatology. 1970;**45**(5):340-345

[38] Lamanna P, Grieco B, Molè R. Preliminary clinical experiences with the topical use of bendazolic acid or bendazac in occupational dermatitis. Minerva Medica. 1979;**61**(24):1201-1208

[39] Fulghesu G, Carta G. Use of a preparation with a bendazolic acid or Bendazac base in occupational dermatitis. Policlinico Medica;**78**(4):170-181

[40] Molinari R. Clinical observations on the local anti-inflammatory action of a new drug (bendazolic acid) in skin diseases in childhood. Clinical Pediatrics (Bologna). 1969;**51**(6):325-337

[41] Caruso F. Therapeutic findings with bendazolic acid in various dermatites in childhood. La Clinica Terapeutica. 1969;**51**(4):363-366

[42] Manfredi G. Use of bendazolic acid in skin diseases in childhood. Clinical Pediatrics (Bologna). 1970;**52**(4):175-181

[43] Silvestrini B, Catanese B, Barillari G, Iorio E, Valeri P. Basic data supporting the use of the l-lysine salt of bendazac in cataract. International Journal of Tissue Reactions. 1983;**5**(2):217-225

[44] Testa M, Iuliano G, Silvestrini B. Pilot study of Bendazac for treatment of cataract. The Lancet 1. 1982:849-850

[45] Balfour JA, Clissold SP, Bendazac lysine. A review of its pharmacological properties and therapeutic potential in the management of cataracts. Drugs. 1990;**39**(4):575-596. DOI: 10.2165/00003495-199039040-00007

[46] Hockwin O, Laser H, De Gregorio M, Carrieri MP. Bendazac lysine in selected types of human senile cataract. A long-term double-masked placebo-controlled clinical trial with multilinear densitometric image analysis of Scheimpflug photographs. Ophthalmic Research. 1989;**21**(3):141-154. DOI: 10.1159/000266799

[47] CioliV, CiarnielloMG, GuglielmottiA, Luparini MR, Durando L, Martinelli B, et al. A new protein antidenaturant agent, bindarit, reduces secondary phase of adjuvant arthritis in rats. The Journal of Rheumatology. 1992;**19**(11):1735-1742

[48] Pearson CM. Development of arthritis, periarthritis and periostitis in rats given adjuvants. Proceedings of the Society for Experimental Biology and Medicine (N.Y.). 1956;**91**:95-101

[49] Waksman BH, Sharp JT. Immunologic nature of arthritis induced in rats by mycobacterial adjuvant. Federation Proceedings. 1960;**19**:210

[50] Newbould BB. Chemotherapy of arthritis induced in rats by mycobacterial adjuvant. British Journal of Pharmacology. 1963;**21**:127-136

[51] Newbould BB. Suppression of adjuvant-induced arthritis in rats with 2-butoxycarbonylmethylene-4-oxothiazolidine. British Journal of Pharmacology and Chemotherapy. 1965;**24**(3):632-640. DOI: 10.1111/j.1476-5381.1965.tb01619.x

[52] Silvestrini B, Natali PG, Catanese B, Barillari G, Cordiali-Fei P. Occurrence of globulin-like migrating blood albumins or GLIMBAL, in pathological rat and human sera. Canadian Journal of Biochemistry. 1980;**58**:89-92

[53] Guglielmotti A, Aquilini L, D'Onofrio E, Rosignoli MT, Milanese C, Pinza M. Bindarit prolongs survival and reduces renal damage in NZB/W lupus mice. Clinical and Experimental Rheumatology. 1998;**16**(2):149-154

[54] Zoja C, Corna D, Benedetti G, Morigi M, Donadelli R, Guglielmotti A, et al. Bindarit retards renal disease and prolongs survival in murine lupus autoimmune disease. Kidney International. 1998;**53**(3):726-734. DOI: 10.1046/j.1523-1755.1998.00804.x

[55] Silvestrini B, Buorberi S, Catanese B. Inflammatory responses in normal and adrenalectomized rats during obstructive jaundice. Japan Journal of Pharmacology. 1968;**18**:421-429

[56] Saso L, Casini ML, Valentini G, Alcaro S, Silvestrini B. Effect of selected substances on heat induced aggregation of albumin examined by HPLC and polyacrylamide gel electrophoresis. Pharmacological Research. 1995;**31**(suppl. 1):214

[57] Saso L, Casini ML, Valentini G, Mattei E, Panzironi C, Silvestrini B. Development of an HPLC assay to study the effect of Endogenous and Exogenous substances on heat-induced aggregation of human serum albumin. Clinical Chemistry and Laboratory Medicine. 1998;**36**(3):155-162

[58] Saso L, Valentini G, Grippa E, Leone MG, Silvestrini B. Effect of selected substances on heat-induced aggregation of albumin, IgG and lysozyme. Research Communications in Molecular Pathology and Pharmacology. 1998;**102**:15-28

[59] Saso L, Valentini G, Casini ML, Mattei E, Braghiroli L, Mazzanti G, et al. Inhibition of protein denaturation by fatty acids, bile salts and other natural substances: A new hypothesis for the mechanism of action of fish oil in rheumatic diseases. Japanese Journal of Pharmacology. 1999;**79**:89-99

[60] Saso L, Valentini G, Mattei E, Panzironi C, Casini ML, Grippa E, et al. Stabilization of rat serum proteins following oral administration of fish oil. Archives of Pharmacal Research. 1999;**22**(5):485-490

[61] Ibarguren M, López DJ, Escribá PV. The effect of natural and synthetic fatty acids on membrane structure, microdomain organization, cellular functions and human health. Biochimica et Biophysica Acta. 2014;**1838**(6):1518-1528. DOI: 10.1016/j.bbamem.2013.12.021

[62] Rybczynska M, Csordas A. Chain length-dependent interaction of free fatty acids with the erythrocyte membrane. Life Sciences. 1989;**44**(9):625-632. DOI: 10.1016/0024-3205(89)90195-1

[63] Catanese B, Lisciani R, Piccinelli D. Erythrocyte membrane stabilization and protein binding of some anti-inflammatory drugs and of deoxycholic acid. Biochemical Pharmacology. 1969;**18**:1707-1710

[64] Ciancarelli-Tozzi MG, Silvestrini B, Finazzi-Agro A. Photosensitized

haemolysis of human erythrocytes is reduced by bendazac. Drugs Under Experimental and Clinical Research. 1989;**15**(5):219-222

[65] Silvestrini B, Cheng CY, Innocenti M. In: Mazumder N, Chakrabarty S, editors. Collagen Involvement in Health, Disease, and Medicine. London: Collagen Biomaterials, IntechOpen; 2022. DOI: 10.5772/intechopen.101978

[66] Silvestrini B, Innocenti M, Perrotta A, Cheng CY. Physiopathology and treatment of collagen carential disease. Minerva Medica. 2021;**112**:403-404. DOI: 10.23736/S0026-4806.19.06036-1

[67] Giulio B. Cento anni di cellule labili, stabili e perenni, di Quaderni dell'Accademia delle scienze di Torino. Vol. 3. Editore Accademia delle scienze di Torino; 1996

[68] Silvestrini B, Medicitali A. Una senescenza sana e longeva. MedicitaliA. 10 maggio; 2022

[69] Walker LC, LeVine H. The cerebral proteopathies. Molecular Neurobiology. 2000;**21**(1):83-95

[70] Stefani M, Dobson CM. Protein aggregation and aggregate toxicity: New insights into protein folding, misfolding diseases and biological evolution. Journal of Molecular Medicine (Berlin, Germany). 2003;**81**(11):678-699. DOI: 10.1007/s00109-003-0464-5

[71] Nilsson SE, Johansson B, Takkinen S, Berg S, Zarit S, McClearn G, et al. Does aspirin protect against Alzheimer's dementia? A study in a Swedish population-based sample aged > or =80 years. European Journal of Clinical Pharmacology. 2003;**59**(4):313-319. DOI: 10.1007/s00228-003-0618-y

Chapter 5

Calcific Tendinitis: Limited Role of Surgery

John Christian Parsaoran Butarbutar

Abstract

Calcific tendinitis is not an uncommon condition, although many patients may experience no symptoms, and calcification was found accidentally through imaging studies. Even so, in some cases, calcific tendinitis may arise with bothersome symptoms that can lead to diminished function of the affected joint. Calcific tendinitis is usually a self-limiting disease, where in its course, it may resolve on its own, may not need further interventions. In symptomatic cases, conservative treatment is the main option. More aggressive treatment such as percutaneous lavage may be needed in acute or unresponsive chronic pain. Surgical intervention may be needed to help resolve the symptoms, but it is rarely indicated.

Keywords: calcified tendinitis, surgery, arthroscopy, ultrasonography, lavage

1. Introduction

Calcific Tendinitis (CT) is a condition of abnormal deposition of calcium salt inside of the tendon. It is also known as calcific periarthritis, which implies that the calcification is not happening within the joint, and calcifying tendinitis, describe the transient nature of the disease [1, 2].

It may occur in many regions of the body, but it is mostly found in the shoulder region, usually the rotator cuff in which the supraspinatus tendon is most frequently affected, followed by the infraspinatus and the subscapularis. Hip girdle region is the second most affected region, including rectus femoris and gluteus Medius tendon. CT also has been reported to occur at proximal hamstring, biceps brachii, longus colli, Achilles, flexor carpi ulnaris, and many other sites [1].

Number of incidences varies between 2.7 to 22% in individuals without symptoms detected by X-Ray with bilateral incidence in about 10–20% of cases [3–5]. A study conducted by Bosworth et al. in 1941 found incidence of 2.7% out of 6061 patients have CT in which 34.7% were symptomatic [4]. A newer descriptive study reported the incidence of calcific tendinosis in the shoulder can be found in 7.8% of asymptomatic patients and 42.5% of patients with subacromial pain syndrome [6]. Both studies have shown that CT affected more women than men, in the age group of 30 to 60.

2. History

Duplay was accredited as the first to describe CT of the shoulder in 1872. He defined it as "painful periarthritis of the shoulder" [7]. Later, Painter rendered the first case report of calcific deposit about the shoulder in 1907, misinterpreting it as thickening of the walls of the bursa [8]. This was followed by other authors who proposed the accumulation of scar tissue [9], hemorrhage under pressure [10] and metamorphosis of fat deposits [11], which suggest subacromial bursa pathology.

In 1908, Codman reported the surgical removal of deposits composed chiefly of calcium, in or on the supraspinatus tendon. In his classic textbook on the shoulder (1934), he then made the following definitive statement: "The deposits do not arise in the bursa itself, but in the tendons beneath it." The critical area, a concept of there being a specific vulnerable area in the supraspinatus tendon susceptible to calcification was first proposed by Codman [12]. Other authors in agreement like Bishop and Sandstrom suggested that some kind of degeneration of the rotator cuff due to overuse or ischemia leads to calcific deposits in the tendon. The process may begin with necrosis of tenocytes along with intracellular accumulation of calcium [13, 14]. This view was then supported by Refior in a later paper, using cadaveric study [15].

In contrast, Uhthoff and Loehr think that the transient, self-healing nature of calcifying tendinitis did not fit the degenerative disease characteristic. They proposed the multiphasic disease theory, which suggests that deposition of calcium in the tissues will be followed by spontaneous resorption of the calcific deposit. They believe that the process of calcification is actively mediated by cells in a viable environment [16]. This view becomes more prevalent in recent years, with imaging studies and classifications adopting different stages of the disease.

Most of our understanding of this disease comes from observation of CT of rotator cuff of the shoulder.

3. Symptoms

CT can present in three different clinical scenarios. It can be an asymptomatic incidental finding, a condition involving chronic low-grade pain, or a very painful acute condition that affects the range of movement and function of the joint. In shoulder, pain is often aggravated by abduction of the arm above shoulder height or by lying on the affected shoulder. Point exquisite tenderness is found in the calcific region, especially in acute phase [17, 18].

4. Investigation

Calcific deposits appear as irregular punctuate, circular, linear, or plaque-like radio-dense areas that do not possess a trabecular or cortical structure. In the rotator cuff tendons, it can be localized using the anteroposterior radiographs of the shoulder in internal and external rotation and axillary lateral radiographs. The French Arthroscopic Society using the anteroposterior view of X-rays which then becomes the widely used classification defined four types of deposits. Type-A calcifications are sharply delineated, dense, and homogenous. Type B are sharply delineated and dense in appearance, with multiple fragments. Type C are heterogeneous in appearance, with a fluffy deposit (**Figure 1**). Type D are dystrophic calcifications at the tendon insertion. The last two types are associated with the resorptive stage of the disease [19, 20].

The second useful investigation is ultrasonographic evaluation. It is sensitive to detecting the calcium deposits in soft tissue. Although in the presence of calcifications, shadows may cause false-positive and false-negative findings, ultrasonographic is still beneficial to detect the cuff tears nearby, and concomitant impingement syndrome. On ultrasound, calcification was classified as arc-shaped (an echogenic arc with clear shadowing), fragmented or punctate (at least 2 separated echogenic spots or plaques) with shadowing, fragmented or punctate without shadowing, and nodular (an echogenic nodule without shadowing) [21]. A study reported that an arc-shaped and hyperechoic deposit indicates calcification in the resting phase, whereas on-arc shaped deposit, may be fragmented, cystic or nodular indicating the resolving phase of the calcification [22]. Bianchi and Martinelo described three types of calcifications based on the percentage of calcium content found by ultrasonography. They described Type I as hyperechoic focci with well-defined acoustic shadowing due to high calcium amount, Type II as hyperechoic focci with mild acoustic shadowing due to reduced calcium amount, and Type III as focci which is isoechoic to the tendon (**Figure 2**) [23].

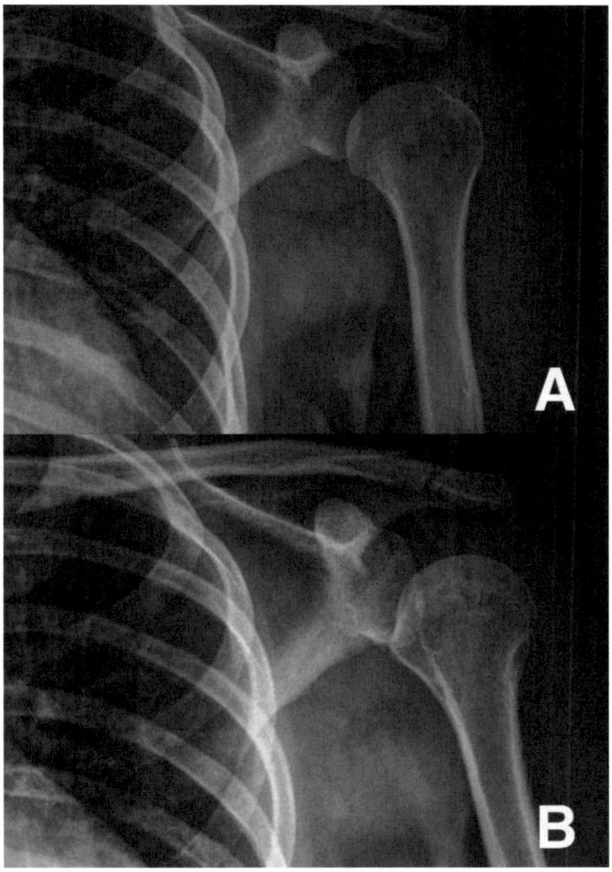

Figure 1.
Anteroposterior (A) and internal rotation (B) view of the left shoulder showing Type C calcification according to French Arthroscopic Association classification within the supraspinatus tendon of a 41-year-old woman.

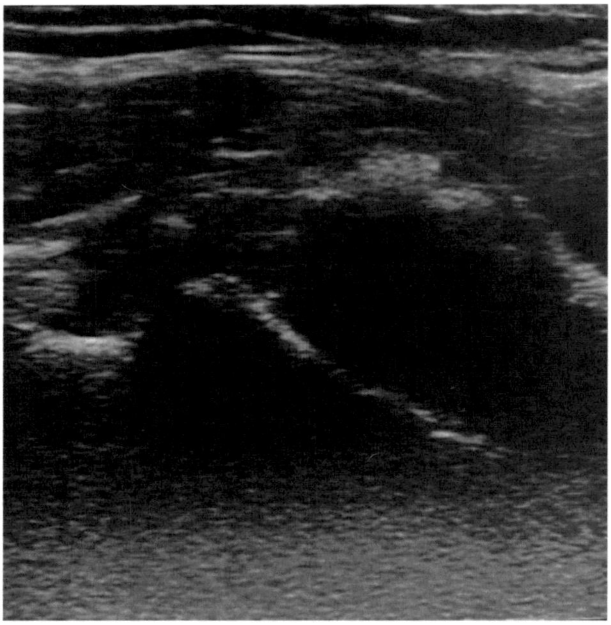

Figure 2.
Ultrasonographic of a 49-year-old woman showed a Type II calcific deposit in the subscapularis tendon according to Bianchi and Martinoli, who later underwent ultrasound-guided percutaneous lavage with dramatic improvement of acute pain.

The use of magnetic resonance imaging in cases of CT has shown to be unessential as it tells no specific additional information and does not alter the treatment plan. The deposit can be found in MRI imaging as a low-intensity lesion in the T1-weighted images. High intensity may be found in T2 sequence indicating edema around the deposit which correlates to the resorptive phase of calcification. MRI also allows better evaluation of coexisting pathology when conservative treatment fails and surgery is indicated [24].

Computed tomography allowed better localization of the deposits but is rarely indicated.

In contrast to metastatic calcification, laboratory findings are usually within normal limits. Some metabolic abnormal findings may be found as a predisposing factor to CT such as type 2 diabetes and hypothyroid conditions [16].

5. Pathomechanism

There are two most accredited proposed mechanisms for CT: degenerative, which highlights similarities with degenerative lesions of the rotator cuff, and reactive, proposed by Uhthoff and Loehr, which suggests that deposition of calcium in the tissues is a cell-mediated process that is followed by spontaneous resorption [15, 16].

The degenerative calcification theory proposes that CT is a form of dystrophic calcification of the tendon that follows an ischemic, degenerative, and necrotic phase, secondary to wear and tear, overuse and microinjury all attributable to aging. In the shoulder, it is suggested that the pathogenesis of both cuff tears and calcific tendinopathy are identical. The concept of there being a specific area in the supraspinatus tendon susceptible to calcification and tearing was first proposed by Codman. This is supported by the observation that CT seldom affects people before the fourth decade [25–27], although studies on correlation between rotator cuff tear and CT showed conflicting results. Another objection is that CT can be observed, not only in the supraspinatus and subscapular tendon within the "avascular critical zone," but also in the subscapularis and teres minor tendon outside the "avascular critical zone".

In contrast, Uhthoff proposed a different mechanism, which is an active calcification followed by resorption and tendon remodeling. The reactive calcification theory involves four phases (pre-calcific, formative, resorptive, and healing). In pre-calcific phase, the fibrocartilaginous focus was developed on extracellular matrix of tendon. Matrix that will be filled with calcium in the calcific phase. In resorptive phase, macrophage and giant cell migrates surrounding the calcification site and begins phagocytosis. In the post-calcific phase, fibroblast proliferation occurs, followed by remodeling of the affected tendon. Uhthoff regards the transformation of fibrocytes into chondrocytes as the initial stage. He was not able to find any similar metaplasia in the case of rotator cuff rupture. Therefore, he concluded that CT and rupture of the rotator cuff have no common degenerative preconditions. The data shows peak at 50 years of age and fail to show that trauma and overuse as risk factor; dominant hand is not more frequent than non-dominant, and it is not more prevalent in heavy jobs. This view is also supported by a variety of imaging studies demonstrating a complete resolution of the calcium deposits. This is confirmed later by several studies [1, 28, 29]. The concept has been challenged by Refior, who was able to prove the simultaneous incidence of rotator cuff ruptures and intra-tendinous calcification in 13 of 22 cases of rotator cuff ruptures. The coexistence of CT and rotator cuff tear is not as rare as previously mentioned. A total of 28%' of patients with CT revealed rotator cuff tear with arthrography study, and five of these were confirmed at surgery [30].

It has been reported in subsequent studies that endocrine disorders (thyroxine, estrogen, insulin) and genetic factors may also be related to the development of CT and affect resolution process.

Long-term data on the natural history of CT vary greatly. Gärtner et al. reported an 85% chance of natural resolution after 3 years for type III deposits, as opposed to 33% for type I and II deposits. In his classic study, Bosworth reported that 6.4% off calcific lesions showed spontaneous resorption.

Neer proposed four types of pain on CT in shoulder. The first type is characterized by pain caused by chemical irritation as a result of the calcium deposits. The second type involves pain caused by increased local pressure within the tissue as it swells. The third type causes impingement-like pain through bursal thickening and irritation by prominent calcium deposits. The fourth type reflects pain caused by chronic stiffness of the glenohumeral joint, such as frozen shoulder [31].

6. Treatment

No treatment is indicated in incidental findings of CT without symptoms.

6.1 Acute stage

This stage represents resorption phase, characterized by acute exquisite focal tenderness with restriction of joint movement, possibly from chemical irritation of calcific deposit. This is associated with The French Arthroscopy Association radiologic type C, with fragmented or nodular appearance on ultrasonography [32]. Although anti-inflammatory drugs, analgesics, and steroid injections had been recommended, ultrasound-guided percutaneous lavage should be the main treatment option, since it has been largely successful in reducing the pain dramatically and removing calcium deposits. ESWT is not feasible because of the associated pain, and there is no indication for more invasive therapeutic measures such as surgery in this stage [33, 34].

6.1.1 Percutaneous lavage of rotator cuff calcific tendinitis (barbotage)

Patients sit whilst putting the affected forelimb behind the back in cases of supra and infraspinatus, and externally rotated in for subscapularis CT. The affected shoulder is facing the operator and the ultrasonography monitor is placed on contralateral side in line with the operator. With aseptic technique, deposits are identified using the Ultrasound linear probe, 12–17 MHz, and entry is made into the deposit, with inline technique, after anesthetizing the pathway. Procedure can be done using large bore needle 18–20G especially if the calcific lesion is hard, or regular 23G needle in cases of soft lesion, with syringe filled with lidocaine. The tip of the needle should be placed at the soft spot of calcific deposit, and the needle should be aimed upward to allow gravity to help facilitate calcific material not returning into the deposit cavity. Some amount of lidocaine is injected by pulsating technique into the lesion, and the dissolved calcium will enter syringe, passively. Repeat injections until the syringe fluid is saturated with the material. Further same procedure continued with saline until no calcific material can be extracted anymore. The puncture and aspiration can be done with 1 or 2 different needles according to preferences. Furthermore, the needle is pulled out slowly until it reaches subdeltoid bursa space, and 20–40 mg triamcinolone mixed with 2 cc lidocaine 2% and 10 cc normal saline is injected. After treatment, the patient is advised to rest his shoulder for several days and avoid above-the-shoulder activity for approximately 3 weeks.

6.2 Chronic stage

Chronic stage of the disease may represent calcific, resorptive, and remodeling phases of the disease. Patient complained of chronic, inconsistent pain that sometimes interferes with daily living and can last for years, especially with shoulder abduction. Tenderness can be felt on the calcific deposit site. Some combined with mechanical impingement pain due to bursal thickening that is best shown with dynamic ultrasonography examination (**Figure 3**).

On newly diagnosed untreated CT with mild symptoms and of radiologic type A, conservative measures such as anti-inflammatory drugs, analgesics, and physiotherapy can be initiated with the aim of stimulating vascularization of the tendon and hence improving the conditions for resorption of the calcium deposit. Subacromial steroid injection could be offered in cases with combined impingement syndrome (**Figure 4**).

In calcification radiologic types A and B, complementary focused ESWT or UGN can be offered to disintegrate the calcium deposit. Both methods had shown clinically significant improvement in function and pain, although UGN shows superiority in calcium resorption [35–37].

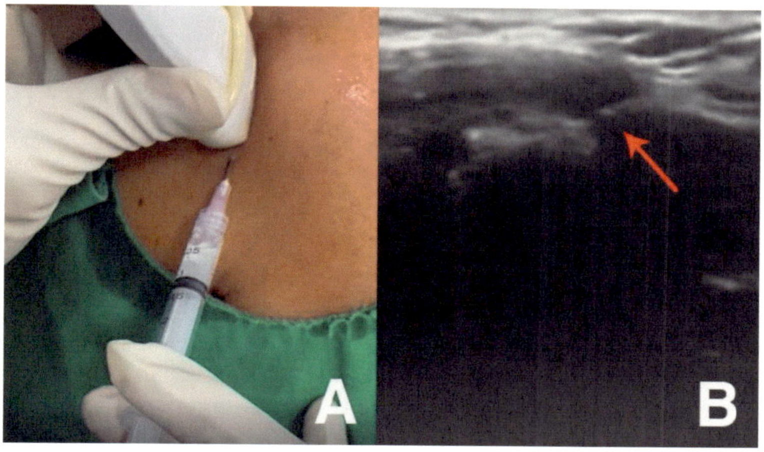

Figure 3.
(A) Clinical image and (B) ultrasonographic image showing needle positioning (red arrow) towards calcium deposit during ultrasound-guided percutaneous lavage of subscapular tendon of the patient from ***Figure 2****, showing saturated syringe content.*

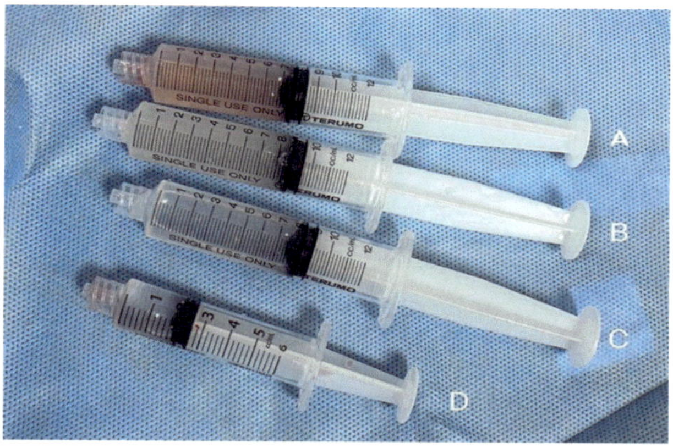

Figure 4.
Post percutaneous lavage shows saturated saline-filled syringes (A), (B), (C) consecutively and (D) saturated lidocaine-filled syringe.

Ultrasonography-guided needling could be repeated after 3 months if the calcific deposit remains, and symptoms persist even if it were previously possible to partially extract the calcium. Finally, steroid injections may be recommended when the calcification has become poorly defined on imaging and it is no longer possible to puncture it. The disappearance of the calcification between 3 and 12 months is also observed in one-third of patients, without any additional treatment [38].

6.2.1 Surgery

Since surgery has a significant risk of iatrogenic tendon tear, it is usually reserved for failed conservative treatment only, especially if it is combined with concomitant lesions such as intraarticular, rotator cuff tear, and impingement syndrome. It consists of open or arthroscopic removal of calcific deposit, with or without tendon repair and decompression with excellent short and mid-term clinical outcomes. But it has shown to have slow recovery of functional scores with majority of patients needing 6 to 12 months to recover [39–42].

6.2.1.1 Arthroscopy removal of calcific deposit

Patient is positioned in either lateral decubitus or beach chair position under general anesthesia, according to the surgeon's preference. Firstly, diagnostic arthroscopy of the glenohumeral joint is performed to address any intra-articular pathology with standard posterior portal. Then, the arthroscope is moved to the subacromial space. A lateral portal is then created above the calcific deposit and bursectomy is performed around the suspected calcific deposit. The calcium deposit is located using probe or by percutaneous needling. Hypervascularization, bulging, or calcific substance might be identified from the bursal site. The overlying tendon is then carefully incised longitudinally using a No. 11 blade and the calcific deposit is then removed by using a probe and motorized shaver. Inaccurate identification of the site of the calcification may result in iatrogenic tendon tears [43]. Intraoperative ultrasound has been reported to increase accuracy of calcific location. The arthroscopic surgery should be converted to mini-open surgery in case of unsuccessful identification of calcific deposit [17].

The surgeon should avoid overzealous calcium deposit removal and should err to incomplete removal to avoid unnecessarily large defects that may be challenging to repair. The remaining tendon after excision of the calcium deposits may not hold the repair. It also may result in excessive tension during margin convergence of the cuff. Although several authors reported shoulder better function in whom complete removal had been achieved [24, 44, 45], recent studies showed that it was not important to remove all the calcific deposit. Residual calcification was resorbed within 6–12 months of the surgical treatment and there were no significant differences in outcomes between patients with and those without complete removal of calcific deposits [39, 40, 42]. The postoperative spontaneous resorption of the remnant calcification may explain the similarity in clinical outcomes between patients whose calcific deposits were completely removed and those whose were not.

Whether it is necessary to repair rotator cuff defect after calcific debridement is debatable. Although rotator cuff repair had been reported to have superior functional outcomes, it had been also related to prolonged recovery [42, 46, 47], and stiffness. Most authors still recommend repairing large defects or encompassing significant thickness of tendon cuff width [48]. That is why surgeon should aim to remove calcific deposit conservatively, using combination of shaver and probe, preserving surrounding healthy tendon as much as possible with longitudinal opening. If large defects resulted despite all efforts, repairing the tendon with side-to-side suture is preferable, which is feasible in majority of cases (**Figure 5**).

6.2.2 Rehabilitation

Since surgery on CT had been shown to have a slow recovery, it is imperative to inform patients before treatment that pain may persist for up to 6 months of the treatment.

No special rehabilitation regimen is prescribed in CT debridement without cuff repair. Several days of rest in a sling are followed by gradual passive and active ROM

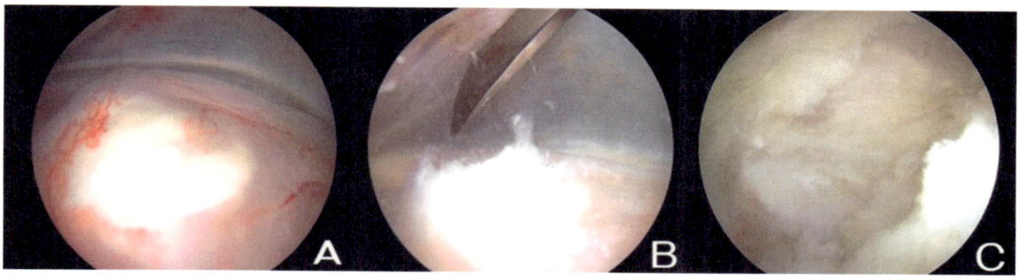

Figure 5.
Subacromial arthroscopic view of (A) supraspinatus calcific tendinitis bulging with hypervascularization on the surface, (B) debridement of calcific deposit, and (C) post debridement.

as tolerated. Patients refrained from excessive load exercises for the first 6 postoperative weeks to avoid disturbance of tendon healing.

In cases with significant defects and cuff repairs, early rehabilitation should be performed to prevent secondary stiffness and shoulder abduction splint is worn for 3 to 6 weeks according to rotator cuff repair protocol [42].

7. Complications

The progression of natural course of untreated disease leads to following complications, although some may also happen postoperatively as well [19].

7.1 Adhesive capsulitis

Adhesive Capsulitis, also known as frozen shoulder can be predisposed by factors inside the shoulder (Fracture, shoulder inflammation, CT) or by extra-articular factors (type 2 diabetes, hyperthyroidism). Some researchers also agree that prolonged immobilization can be a factor predisposing adhesive capsulitis [49, 50]. In symptomatic cases of CT, the calcification may cause severe pain and therefore may induce voluntary immobility. In cases of chronic CT, pain may have subsided, but limited range of shoulder motion is almost always noted, in which adhesive capsulitis becomes the common sequela. On another hand, adhesive capsulitis may be associated with the inflammation that's happening within the surrounding structures of the shoulder, and as previously mentioned, systemic diseases such as diabetes can be a predisposing factor to both CT and adhesive capsulitis. A study done by Jacobs et al. also showed that 18% of patients who underwent arthroscopy removal of the calcification experienced adhesive capsulitis and was suggested due to irritation of shoulder capsule by the residual calcium debris [51].

7.2 Greater tuberosity osteolysis

Greater tuberosity osteolysis is one of the rare complications of CT. A study done by Porcellini et al. shows that calcium deposits that come in contact with the tuberosities have consistently caused cortical lesions. This cortical lesion that happens due to biochemical effects of bone lysis can lead to insertion of calcification into the bone, which may cause further pain [52].

7.3 Ossifying tendinitis

Ossifying tendinitis is also a rare complication of CT. Ossifying tendinitis usually happens due to trauma or surgical intervention in the Achilles tendon, gluteus maximus tendon, and distal biceps. A case series and literature review by Merolla et al. found ossifying tendinitis histologically when performed a CT arthroscopy removal. Two cases were described showing persistent shoulder pain that was previously diagnosed as CT, but when removal was done, the calcification was found to be hard. Histological examination showed bone metaplasia. It was hypothesized that ossification happened because of mesenchymal cell transformation to bone-forming cells as a result of the calcification excision previously done [53].

8. Conclusion

Although CT is a transient disease that has self-healing nature, it can result in severe acute or prolonged chronic pain. X-ray, and ultrasonography are the most essential investigation for diagnosis and treatment plans. Conservative treatment should be the main treatment in newly diagnosed CT with mild symptoms, but more aggressive treatment is frequently needed in acute phase or unresponsive chronic phase. Ultrasound-guided percutaneous needling and lavage had been shown to effectively reduce pain and remove calcific deposits. It can be repeated in the less-responsive cases. Surgery role is limited. It should be reserved only for failed conservative treatment. Preservation of surrounding living tissue of the calcification during debridement should be a priority since residual calcification from incomplete excision can be resorbed spontaneously.

Acknowledgements

We thank Earlene Tasya Suginawan, MD for the assistance with English redaction and references that greatly improved the manuscript. We also thank Troydimas Panjaitan, MD for letting us use his arthroscopy images.

Conflict of interest

The authors declare no conflict of interest.

Author details

John Christian Parsaoran Butarbutar
Faculty of Medicine Universitas Pelita Harapan, Department of Orthopaedic and Traumatology, Tangerang, Indonesia

*Address all correspondence to: john.butarbutar@lecturer.uph.edu

References

[1] Beckmann NM. Calcium apatite deposition disease: Diagnosis and treatment. Radiology Research and Practice. 2016;**2016**:1-16

[2] Uhthoff HK, Sarkar K. Calcifying tendinitis. Baillière's Clinical Rheumatology. 1989;**3**(3):567-581

[3] Ogon P, Suedkamp NP, Jaeger M, Izadpanah K, Koestler W, Maier D. Prognostic factors in nonoperative therapy for chronic symptomatic calcific tendinitis of the shoulder. Arthritis and Rheumatism. 2009;**60**(10):2978-2984

[4] Bosworth BM. Calcium deposits in the shoulder and subacromial bursitis: A survey of 12,122 shoulders. Journal of the American Medical Association. 1941;**116**(22):2477-2481

[5] DePalma AF, Kruper JS. Long-term study of shoulder joints afflicted with and treated for calcific tendinitis. Clinical Orthopaedics. 1961;**20**:61-72

[6] Louwerens JKG, Sierevelt IN, van Hove RP, van den Bekerom MPJ, van Noort A. Prevalence of calcific deposits within the rotator cuff tendons in adults with and without subacromial pain syndrome: Clinical and radiologic analysis of 1219 patients. Journal of Shoulder and Elbow Surgery. 2015;**24**(10):1588-1593. Available from. DOI: 10.1016/j.jse.2015.02.024

[7] Duplay S. About periarthritis scapulothoracalis and the resulting painful shoulder [in French]. Archives of General Internal Medicine. 1872;**513**:542

[8] Painter C. Subdeltoid bursitis. Boston Medical and Surgical Journal. 1907;**156**:345-349

[9] Baer WS. Operative treatment of subdeltoid bursitis. Bulletin of the Johns Hopkins Hospital. 1907;**18**:282-285

[10] Brickner WM. Prevalent fallagies concerning suba cromial bursitis. its pathogenesis and rational operative treatment. The American Journal of the Medical Sciences. 1915;**149**(3):351-364

[11] Stern WG. Metamorphosed fat deposits in subdeltoid bursitis. Surgery, Gynecology and Obstetrics. 1925;**40**:92-94

[12] Codman EA. The Shoulder: Rupture of the Supraspinatus Tendon and Other Lesions in or About the Subacromial Bursa. The Shoulder. Boston; 1934. pp. 1869-1940

[13] Bishop WA. Calcification of the supraspinatus tendon: Cause, pathologic picture and relation to the scalenus anticus syndrome. Archives of Surgery. 1939;**39**(2):231-246. Available from. DOI: 10.1001/archsurg.1939.012001400 63006

[14] Sandstrom AC. Peritendinitis calcarea; a common disease of middle life; diagnosis, pathology, and treatment. The American Journal of Roentgenology RADIUM Therapy and Nuclear Medicine. 1938;**40**:1-21

[15] Refior HJ, Krödel A, Melzer C. Examinations of the pathology of the rotator cuff. Archives of Orthopaedic and Trauma Surgery. 1987;**106**(5): 301-308. Available from. DOI: 10.1007/ BF00454338

[16] Uhthoff HK, Loehr JW. Calcific tendinopathy of the rotator cuff: Pathogenesis, diagnosis, and management. Journal of the

American Academy of Orthopaedic Surgeons. 1997;5(4). Available from: https://journals.lww.com/jaaos/Fulltext/1997/07000/Calcific_Tendinopathy_of_the_Rotator_Cuff_.1.aspx

[17] Catapano M, Robinson DM, Schowalter S, Mcinnis KC. Clinical evaluation and management of calcific tendinopathy: An evidence-based review. Journal of Osteopathic Medicine. 2022;**122**(3):141-151

[18] de Carli A, Pulcinelli F, Rose GD, Pitino D, Ferretti A. Calcific tendinitis of the shoulder. Joints. 2004;**2**(3):130-136

[19] Merolla G, Bhat MG, Paladini P, Porcellini G. Complications of calcific tendinitis of the shoulder: A concise review. Journal of Orthopaedics and Traumatology. 2015;**16**(3):175-183. Available from. DOI: 10.1007/s10195-015-0339-x

[20] Molé D, Kempf JF, Gleyze P, Rio B, Bonnomet F, Walch G. Results of endoscopic treatment of non-broken tendinopathies of the rotator cuff. 2. Calcifications of the rotator cuff. Revue de Chirurgie Orthopédique et Réparatrice de l'Appareil Moteur. 1993;**79**(7):532-541. Available from: http://europepmc.org/abstract/MED/8085035

[21] Chiou H-J, Chou Y-H, Wu J-J, Hsu C-C, Huang D-Y, Chang C-Y. Evaluation of calcific tendonitis of the rotator cuff. Journal of Ultrasound in Medicine. 2002;**21**(3):289-295. Available from. DOI: 10.7863/jum.2002.21.3.289

[22] Lin CH, Chao HL, Chiou HJ. Calcified plaque resorptive status as determined by high-resolution ultrasound is predictive of successful conservative management of calcific tendinosis. European Journal of Radiology. 2012;**81**(8):1776-1781

[23] Bianchi S, Martinoli C. Shoulder. In: Ultrasound of the Musculoskeletal System. Berlin: Springer; 2007. pp. 198-332

[24] Merolla G, Singh S, Paladini P, Porcellini G. Calcific tendinitis of the rotator cuff: State of the art in diagnosis and treatment. Journal of Orthopaedics and Traumatology. 2016;**17**(1):7-14

[25] Rathburn JB, Macnab I. The microvascular pattern of the rotator cuff. The Journal of Bone and Joint Surgery. 1970;**52B**(3):540-553

[26] Booth RE, Marvel JP. Differential diagnosis of shoulder pain. Orthopedic Clinics of North America. 1975;**6**(2):353-379. Available from: https://www.sciencedirect.com/science/article/pii/S0030589820310038

[27] Riley GP, Harrall RL, Constant CR, Chard MD, Cawston TE, Hazleman BL. Tendon degeneration and chronic shoulder pain: Changes in the collagen composition of the human rotator cuff tendons in rotator cuff tendinitis. Annals of the Rheumatic Diseases. 1994;53(6):359-366. Available from: http://ard.bmj.com/content/53/6/359.abstract

[28] Yu XK, Li J, Zhang L, Li L, Li JX, Guo WB. Magnetic resonance imaging evaluation of the correlation between calcific tendinitis and rotator cuff injury. BMC Medical Imaging. [Internet]. 2022;**22**(1):1-9. DOI: 10.1186/s12880-022-00746-0

[29] Compagnoni R, Menon A, Radaelli S, Lanzani F, Gallazzi MB, Tassi A, et al. Long - term evolution of calcific tendinitis of the rotator cuff: Clinical and radiological evaluation 10 years after diagnosis. Journal of Orthopaedics and Traumatology. 2021;**22**(1):42-51. Available from. DOI: 10.1186/s10195-021-00604-9

[30] Hsu H, Wu J, Jim Y. Calcific tendinitis and rotator cuft tearing: A clinical and radiographic study. Journal of Shoulder and Elbow Surgery. 1994;**3**(3):159-164. Available from. DOI: 10.1016/S1058-2746(09)80095-5

[31] Neer CI. Less frequent procedures. In: CSE N II, editor. Shoulder Reconstruction. Philadephia, PA: WB Saunders; 1990

[32] Kim M, Kim I, Lee S, Shin S. Diagnosis and treatment of calcific tendinitis of the shoulder. Clinics in Shoulder and Elbow. 2020;**23**(4):210-216

[33] Chiou H-J, Chou Y-H, Wu J-J, Huang T-F, Ma H-L, Hsu C-C, et al. The role of high-resolution ultrasonography in management of calcific tendonitis of the rotator cuff. Ultrasound in Medicine & Biology. 2001;**27**(6):735-743

[34] McKendry RJ, Uhthoff HK, Sarkar K, Hyslop PS. Calcifying tendinitis of the shoulder: Prognostic value of clinical, histologic, and radiologic features in 57 surgically treated cases. The Journal of Rheumatology. 1982;**9**(1):75-80

[35] de Witte PB, Selten JW, Navas A, Nagels J, Visser CPJ, Nelissen RGHH, et al. Calcific tendinitis of the rotator cuff: A randomized controlled trial of ultrasound-guided needling and lavage versus subacromial corticosteroids. The American Journal of Sports Medicine. 2013;**41**(7):1665-1673. Available from. DOI: 10.1177/0363546513487066

[36] Kim Y-S, Lee H-J, Kim Y, Kong C-G. Which method is more effective in treatment of calcific tendinitis in the shoulder? Prospective randomized comparison between ultrasound-guided needling and extracorporeal shock wave therapy. Journal of Shoulder and Elbow Surgery. 2014;23(11):1640-1646. Available from: https://www.sciencedirect.com/science/article/pii/S1058274614003383

[37] Louwerens JKG, Sierevelt IN, Kramer ET, Boonstra R, van den Bekerom MPJ, van Royen BJ, et al. Comparing ultrasound-guided needling combined with a subacromial corticosteroid injection versus high-energy extracorporeal shockwave therapy for calcific tendinitis of the rotator cuff: A randomized controlled trial. Arthroscopy The Journal of Arthroscopic and Related Surgery. 2020;36(7):1823-1833.e1. Available from: https://www.sciencedirect.com/science/article/pii/S0749806320301821

[38] Dumoulin N, Cormier G, Varin S, Coiffier G, Albert J-D, Le Goff B, et al. Factors associated with clinical improvement and the disappearance of calcifications after ultrasound-guided percutaneous lavage of rotator cuff calcific tendinopathy: A post hoc analysis of a randomized controlled trial. The American Journal of Sports Medicine. 2021;**49**(4):883-891. Available from. DOI: 10.1177/03635465 21992359

[39] Seil R, Litzenburger H, Kohn D, Rupp S. Arthroscopic treatment of chronically painful calcifying tendinitis of the supraspinatus tendon. Arthroscopy: The Journal of Arthroscopic & Related Surgery. 2006;**22**(5):521-527

[40] Maier D, Jaeger M, Izadpanah K, Bornebusch L, Suedkamp NP, Ogon P. Rotator cuff preservation in arthroscopic treatment of calcific tendinitis. Arthroscopy: The Journal of Arthroscopic & Related Surgery. 2013;**29**(5):824-831

[41] Lee S, Physiotherapy BAS, Cheng B, Physiotherapy BAS, Grimmer-somers K. The midterm effectiveness of

extracorporeal shockwave therapy in the management of chronic calcific shoulder tendinitis. Journal of Shoulder and Elbow Surgery. 2011;**20**(5):845-854. Available from. DOI: 10.1016/j.jse.2010.10.024

[42] Cho C, Bae K, Kim B, Kim H, Kim D. Recovery pattern after arthroscopic treatment for calcific tendinitis of the shoulder. Orthopaedics & Traumatology: Surgery & Research. 2020;**106**(4):687-691. Available from. DOI: 10.1016/j.otsr.2020.03.005

[43] Morsy MG, Taha Waly AH, Galal MA, Mohamed Ayman EH, Gawish HM. Arthroscopic excision of infraspinatus calcific tendinitis with double-row margin convergence repair. Arthroscopy Techniques. 2021;10(6):e1455–e1467. Available from: https://www.sciencedirect.com/science/article/pii/S2212628721000669

[44] Burkhart SS, Tehrany AM. Arthroscopic subscapularis tendon repair: Technique and preliminary results. The Journal of Arthroscopic and Related Surgery. 2002;**18**(5):454-463

[45] Jerosch J, Strauss M, Schmiel S, Munchen D. Arthroscopic treatment of calcific tendinitis of the shoulder. Journal of Shoulder and Elbow Surgery. 1998;7(1):30-37

[46] Balke M, Bielefeld R, Schmidt C, Dedy N, Liem D. Calcifying tendinitis of the shoulder midterm results after arthroscopic treatment. The American Journal of Sports Medicine. 2012;**40**(3):657-661

[47] Korolev AV, Ilyin DO, Frolov AV, Ryazantsev MS, Magnitskaya NE, Burtsev ME, et al. Outcomes of surgical repair of partial thickness rotator cuff tears in patients with calcific tendinitis. Genij Ortopedii. 2019;**25**(4):452-459

[48] Lee TK, Shin S. Functional recovery of the shoulder after arthroscopic treatment for chronic calcific tendinitis. Clinics in Shoulder and Elbow. 2018;**21**(2):75-81

[49] Kim DH, Lee KH, Lho YM, Ha E, Hwang I, Song KS, et al. Characterization of a frozen shoulder model using immobilization in rats. Journal of Orthopaedic Surgery and Research. 2016;**11**(1):1-6. Available from. DOI: 10.1186/s13018-016-0493-8

[50] Le HV, Lee SJ, Nazarian A, Rodriguez EK. Adhesive capsulitis of the shoulder: Review of pathophysiology and current clinical treatments. Shoulder Elbow. 2017;**9**(2):75-84

[51] Jacobs R, Debeer P. Calcifying tendinitis of the rotator cuff: Functional outcome after arthroscopic treatment. Acta Orthopaedica Belgica. 2006;**72**(3):276-281

[52] Porcellini G, Paladini P, Campi F. Osteolytic lesion of greater tuberosity in calcific tendinitis of the shoulder. Journal of Shoulder and Elbow Surgery. 2009;**18**(2):210-215. Available from. DOI: 10.1016/j.jse.2008.09.016

[53] Merolla G, Dave AC, Paladini P, Campi F, Porcellini G. Ossifying tendinitis of the rotator cuff after arthroscopic excision of calcium deposits: Report of two cases and literature review. Journal of Orthopaedics and Traumatology. 2015;**16**(1):67-73